GLYCEMIC LOAD
FOOD GUIDE

&

PERSONAL WORKBOOK

GLYCEMIC LOAD
FOOD GUIDE

&

PERSONAL WORKBOOK

By

Judith Lickus BSc, LBSW

JML Publishing

Corpus Christi, TX, USA 78404

Notice

This book is sold with the understanding that the author is not liable for the misconception or misuse of any information provided. The information presented here is in no way intended as a substitute for medical treatment or nutritional counseling.

Links to internet resources are current at time of publication.

TABLE OF CONTENTS

OVERVIEW

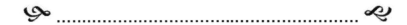

- <u>Cancer</u> – With over 100 types of cancer, the American Cancer Society estimates that when statistics are compiled for 2019, 1,762,450 cases will be newly diagnosed, and nearly 606,880 people will die of cancer. And these numbers are growing every year. But they're not talking about:
  - o Eating certain types of foods are related to a 69% reduction in breast cancer
  - o Men who ate 4 specific foods had an 89% greater chance of developing prostate cancer.

- <u>Coronary Heart Disease</u> (CHD) – This silent but deadly killer is responsible for about one in every four deaths (25%). It takes the lives of one out of every three women (33.3%). Learn more about the subtle symptoms and complications at the <u>National Institutes of Health</u>.

- <u>Depression</u> – According to the World Health Organization, in 2019, over 264 million worldwide suffered depression, with over 800,000 suicides. In the U.S., 17.3 million or 7.1% of the adult population had a <u>major depressive episode</u> over the past year.
  - o Certain foods are related to a 55% higher score for Total Mood Disturbance

- <u>Type 2 diabetes</u> – According to the Center for Disease Control, diabetes is up 800% from 1960 to the present. Over 30.3 million, or about 9.4% of the U.S. population has diabetes. Prediabetes affects 84.1 million or nearly 34% of Americans.
  - o Nearly 24% of people with diabetes are undiagnosed.
  - o One of every ten people twenty 20 yrs. and older have diabetes.
  - o For those 65 and older the figure rises to one in four.

Most diseases and disorders are the byproducts, the outcomes of the way we have lived our lives for many years. We came into this world to live long and healthy lives. And the beauty is that science has demonstrated the links between *how* we live and how healthy we remain. They call these links "associations." Understanding these associations puts us in a position to take action. Let's take a closer look at some associations right now.

PART 1: THE ASSOCIATIONS

᠙ .... ᡖ

CANCER

When we speak of "associations," we are looking for a connection, a relationship, or a link. Let's look at the association between cigarette smoking and lung cancer deaths. The following diagram by Sakurambo plots the "association" or link between lung cancer deaths and cigarette smoking:

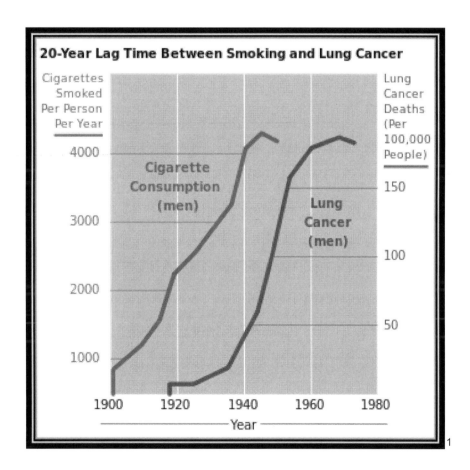

[1] <a title="Sakurambo / Public domain" href="https://commons.wikimedia.org/wiki/File:Cancer_smoking_lung_cancer_correlation_from_NIH.svg"><img width="256" alt="Cancer smoking lung cancer correlation from NIH" rc="https://upload.wikimedia.org/wikipedia/commons/thumb/9/94/Cancer_smoking_lung_cancer_correlation_from_NIH.svg/256px-Cancer_smoking_lung_cancer_correlation_from_NIH.svg.png"></a>

Notice there is a lag time of 20 years between the smoking behavior and the onset of lung cancer. You may also notice that the number of cigarettes smoked is *associated* with increased frequency of lung cancer.

Do you think we can say that there is essentially conclusive evidence that cigarette smoking is "associated" with lung cancer?

Remember how the tobacco industry long maintained that smoking and lung cancer were unrelated?

In June, 2013 a panel of carbohydrate metabolism experts gathered on a little island off the coast of Italy. After reviewing current scientific data, they expressed an urgent need to communicate information on GI and GL to the general public and health professionals, through channels such as national dietary guidelines, food composition tables and food labels. They said this because they claim that they saw essentially conclusive evidence that high GI/GL diets contribute to risk of T2DM and CVD [cardio-vascular disease].

They went on to say that they saw moderate to weak associations for selected cancers. Those cancers included breast, colorectal, endometrial, and prostate. Here is what they said: "Dietary carbohydrates increase blood glucose and insulin concentrations at different rates and levels depending on their GI …. Insulin acts as a growth factor increasing the bioactivity of the cancer-promoting insulin-like growth factor-1 (IGF-1) which has proliferatory, angiogenic, anti-apoptotic and estrogen-stimulating properties.

It has been proposed that low GI foods by virtue of their lower glucose rises and overall insulin economy may beneficially influence cancer risk compared to high GI foods." [2]

They also reported some unexpected findings.

---

[2] Nutrition, Metabolism & Cardiovascular Diseases
September 2015Volume 25, Issue 9, Pages 795–815
Accessed 10-04-16 at: http://www.nmcd-journal.com/article/S0939-4753(15)00127-1/fulltext#tbl1
DOI: http://dx.doi.org/10.1016/j.numecd.2015.05.005
Based on the meeting "Glycemic Index, Glycemic Load and Glycemic Response: an International Scientific Consensus Summit" held in Stresa (Italy) on June 6–7th, 2013.
Authors of the section: La Vecchia C. and Augustin L., "GI/GL and risk of major cancers: what can we conclude based on epidemiological evidence?" Section F of Article outline.

NEVER SMOKERS AND LUNG CANCER

Dietary glycemic index (GI) is also separately associated with lung cancer risk in *non-smokers*, according to a study published in the March, 2016 issue of *"Cancer Epidemiology, Biomarkers & Prevention"*.[3]

The authors of the study looked at GI, GL, and lung cancer risk.

They reviewed dietary GI and GL data for 1,905 newly diagnosed lung cancer cases from the MD Anderson Cancer Center in Houston, TX.

They report that "Postprandial glucose (PPG) and insulin responses play a role in carcinogenesis… We observed a significant association between GI and lung cancer risk. We observed a more pronounced association between GI and lung cancer risk among never smokers."[4]

CANCER AND GLYCEMIC LOAD

In 2015, the Journal of Molecular Nutrition & Food Research published a systematic review and meta-analysis performed by researchers to determine if the glycemic index and glycemic load had any influence on the incidence of cancer. The researchers reviewed seventy-five reports on over one hundred forty-seven thousand cases. That is a lot of cases. Their conclusions: "High-GI and high-GL diets are related to moderately increased risk of cancer at several common sites."[5]

In 2016, The *American Cancer Society* (ACS) decided to take a closer look at the "moderately increased risk of cancer at several common sites". They looked specifically at the associations of the specific *types* of carbohydrate consumed, glycemic index, glycemic load, and cancer.

[3] Practice Update. Accessed 10-03-16 at: http://www.practiceupdate.com/content/dietary-glycemic-index-linked-to-lung-cancer-risk/36354

[4] Melkonian S, Daniel C, Ye Y, et al. "Glycemic Index, Glycemic Load, and Lung Cancer Risk in Non-Hispanic Whites." American Association for Cancer Research: Cancer Epidemiology, Biomarkers & Prevention. Published March 2016 DOI: 10.1158/1055-9965.EPI-15-0765
Accessed 10-03-16 at: http://cebp.aacrjournals.org/content/25/3/532

[5] Turati F, Galeone C, Gandini S, et al. "High glycemic index and glycemic load are associated with moderately increased cancer risk." Mol Nutr Food Res. 2015 Jul; 59(7):1384-94. Doi: 10.1002/mnfr.201400594.
https://www.ncbi.nlm.nih.gov/pubmed/25693843
Epub 2015 Apr 2.
Accessed 10-02-16 at: https://www.ncbi.nlm.nih.gov/pubmed/25693843

Results of the ACS research were first available in April, 2016 as an abstract from the Experimental Biology 2016 Meeting. The *Federation of American Societies of Experimental Biology* published this abstract in their journal.[6]

You'll see some of their findings presented in the numbered list following this text from their abstract:

"The aim of this prospective cohort study is to investigate the role of dietary carbohydrates, glycemic index (GI) and glycemic load (GL) in the risk of adiposity-related cancers combined and three of the most commonly diagnosed site-specific cancers: breast, prostate and colorectal.

The study sample consisted of 3,184 men and women from the Framingham Offspring cohort recruited in 1971–1975. The researchers of this study followed these 3,184 participants from 1991 to 2013, longer than a 20 year period. (Even though the accumulation of study data began in 1971, the data on the diets of these subjects only first became available in 1991.)

Additionally, individuals included in the study identified specific major carbohydrate food sources in their diet by using the Continuing Survey of Food Intakes by Individuals. Using the American Diabetes Association (ADA) definition,[7] high, medium and low GI foods were categorized."[8]

The study focus areas were combined incidence of all adiposity-related cancers and first primary incidence of breast, prostate and colorectal cancers. Cancers were considered adiposity-related if identified by the National Cancer Institute as clearly or possibly linked to overweight and obesity.[9]

Doctor-diagnosed cancers were documented using medical records (n=565) until 2013. The study period, from 1991 to 2013, represents a follow-up of over 20 years. Cox proportional hazards models were used to compute hazard ratios (HR) and 95% confidence intervals (CI) to estimate associations between dietary carbohydrates, *their major food sources*, GI, GL and cancer risk.

SPECIFIC CANCERS RELATED TO SPECIFIC FOODS

---

[6] Makarem N, Lin Y, Bandera E. "Dietary Carbohydrate Intake, Glycemic Index and Glycemic Load in Relation to Adiposity-Related Cancer Risk: Results from The Framingham Offspring Cohort (1991–2013)." April 2016 The FASEB Journal vol. 30 no. 1 Supplement 417.7 Accessed at: http://www.fasebj.org/content/30/1_Supplement/417.7

[7] https://www.diabetes.org/glycemic-index-and-diabetes

[8] Retrieved on 4-21--20 from: https://www.diabetes.org/glycemic-index-and-diabetes

[9] https://www.cancer.gov/about-cancer/causes-prevention/risk/obesity/obesity-fact-sheet

Here are the findings from this Framingham Offspring Cohort study:

1. "Higher GL was associated with a 78% higher risk of prostate cancer.
2. Among food sources, consumption of low GI foods was associated with a 69% reduction in breast cancer risk.
3. Among individual foods, legumes were associated with 35% lower adiposity-related cancer risk.
4. While lunch foods (pizza, burgers, meat sandwiches and casseroles) were associated with 89% higher prostate cancer risk.
5. Among beverages, consumption of soft drinks and fruit juice was associated >3-fold higher risk of prostate cancer."[10]

Let's try to restate a couple of these findings in more positive terms as we take a closer look the three prostate cancer associations noted above:

1. 22% of men eating a high GL diet did not get prostate cancer.
2. 11% of men eating pizza, burgers, meat sandwiches and casserole lunches did not get prostate cancer.
3. Only the men who (by their own reports) added a soft drink or fruit juice to their meal -- tripled their risk for prostate cancer.

Even while they were unaware, it's a lot like these men were trying to catch a falling knife … between their thighs.

CORONARY HEART DISEASE (CHD)

STROKE – A CEREBROVASCULAR ACCIDENT

With over 200,000 diagnosed cases a year, stroke is a major cerebrovascular accident that damages the brain. There are two basic types of stroke, ischemic (clots) and hemorrhagic (bleeds). Both create a blockage in blood flow to the brain.

According to the American Heart Association/American Stroke Association, Ischemic stroke (caused by a blood clot) accounts for about 87% of all cases of stroke.[11] Ischemic strokes occur as a result of an obstruction within a blood

---

[10] Makarem N, Lin Y, Bandera E. "Dietary Carbohydrate Intake, Glycemic Index and Glycemic Load in Relation to Adiposity-Related Cancer Risk: Results from The Framingham Offspring Cohort (1991–2013)." April 2016 The FASEB Journal vol. 30 no. 1 Supplement 417.7 Accessed at: http://www.fasebj.org/content/30/1_Supplement/417.7

vessel supplying blood to the brain. "The underlying condition for this type of obstruction is the development of fatty deposits lining the vessel walls. This condition is called atherosclerosis."[12] You can watch a video here.[13] Or you can visit the link in the footnotes.

Atherosclerosis is a very common disease, with more than 3 million newly diagnosed cases a year in the US alone. "Arteriosclerosis occurs when the blood vessels (arteries) that carry oxygen and nutrients from your heart to the rest of your body become thick and stiff — sometimes restricting blood flow to your organs and tissues.

Healthy arteries are flexible and elastic, but over time, the walls in your arteries can harden, a condition commonly called "hardening of the arteries."

Atherosclerosis is a specific type of arteriosclerosis, but the terms are sometimes used interchangeably. Atherosclerosis refers to the buildup of fats, cholesterol and other substances in and on your artery walls (plaques), which can also restrict blood flow.

These plaques can burst, triggering a blood clot. Although atherosclerosis is often considered a heart problem, it can affect arteries anywhere in your body. According to the Mayo Clinic, atherosclerosis may be preventable and is treatable." [14]

Prevention and treatment are only possible when you know what to do. Remember what the glycemic researchers said at the Glycemic Summit, "Overall, the dietary GI seems to be the strongest risk factor for T2DM while GL for heart disease." [15] Let's take a closer look at how the GL affects the state of our cardiovascular health.

[11] http://www.strokeassociation.org/STROKEORG/AboutStroke/TypesofStroke/IschemicClots/Ischemic-Strokes-Clots_UCM_310939_Article.jsp#.WDtAAuSQzlU Accessed 11-27-16
[12] Ibid.
[13] http://watchlearnlive.heart.org/CVML_Player.php?moduleSelect=iscstr Accessed 11-27-16
[14] http://www.mayoclinic.org/diseases-conditions/arteriosclerosis-atherosclerosis/home/ovc-20167019 Accessed 11-27-16
[15] Augustin L, Kendall C, Jenkins D, et al. "Glycemic index, glycemic load and glycemic response: An International Scientific Consensus Summit from the International Carbohydrate Quality Consortium (ICQC)." Nutr Metab Cardiovasc Dis. 2015 Sep; 25(9):795-815. Doi: 10.1016/j.numecd.2015.05.005. Epub 2015 May 16.
Abstract Accessed 10-02-16 at: https://www.ncbi.nlm.nih.gov/pubmed/26160327
Full text document accessed 10-04-16 at: http://www.nmcd-journal.com/article/S0939-4753(15)00127-1/fulltext

HDL LEVELS

A study, published in 2007 by the *Journal of the American Medical Association* (JAMA), highlights the importance of the glycemic load in high density lipoprotein (HDL) levels. Researchers compared the effects of a low glycemic load vs a low fat diet in obese young adults. They report that: "Reducing glycemic load may be especially important to achieve weight loss among individuals with high insulin secretion."[16]

Higher amounts of HDL particles (the good ones) are strongly *associated* with decreasing accumulations of atherosclerosis within arterial walls. That's because HDL particles remove fat molecules such as cholesterol, phospholipids, and triglycerides from cells. "This is important because atherosclerosis eventually results in sudden plaque ruptures, cardiovascular disease, stroke and other vascular diseases." [17]

In the above JAMA study, the authors go on to explain that "Regardless of insulin secretion, a low–glycemic load diet has beneficial effects on high-density lipoprotein [HDL] cholesterol and triglyceride concentrations but not on low-density lipoprotein [LDL] cholesterol concentration."[18]

Isn't HDL what protects your heart from coronary heart disease? We wondered how strong the relationship might be between low GL recipes and CHD. We wondered how quickly the body would respond to this sweeping away of cholesterol, phospholipids, and triglycerides from the arterial walls. What would that look like? Is this something that we can measure? How fast will a change occur?

Volunteers eager to turn the tide on their own low HDL/high LDL levels, tested the low glycemic load recipes being prepared for the book *"Low Glycemic Happiness: 120 Recipes for Blood Sugar Control,"* published in 2014. (This was long before the "Special Communication" about the sugar industry was reported. As you read on, the upcoming chapter "Sweet Deception..." details this "Special Communication" thoroughly.) But back in 2014, one individual proudly shared a digital file of HDL blood test results after three months of

---

[16] Ebbeling C, Leidig M, Feldman H, et al. Effects of a Low–Glycemic Load vs Low-Fat Diet in Obese Young Adults. JAMA. 2007; 297(19):2092-2102. doi:10.1001/jama.297.19.2092.
Accessed 10-04-16 at: http://jama.jamanetwork.com/article.aspx?articleid=207088

[17] https://en.wikipedia.org/wiki/High-density_lipoprotein Accessed 11-27-16

[18] Ebbeling C, Leidig M, Feldman H, et al. Effects of a Low–Glycemic Load vs Low-Fat Diet in Obese Young Adults. JAMA. 2007; 297(19):2092-2102. doi:10.1001/jama.297.19.2092.
Accessed 10-04-16 at: http://jama.jamanetwork.com/article.aspx?articleid=207088

eating the low glycemic load recipes in the book.

In the image below, you can see what just three months of a low glycemic load lifestyle did for HDL levels. It was a surprise because this "innocent" side effect was not yet recognized through publication in the scientific community:

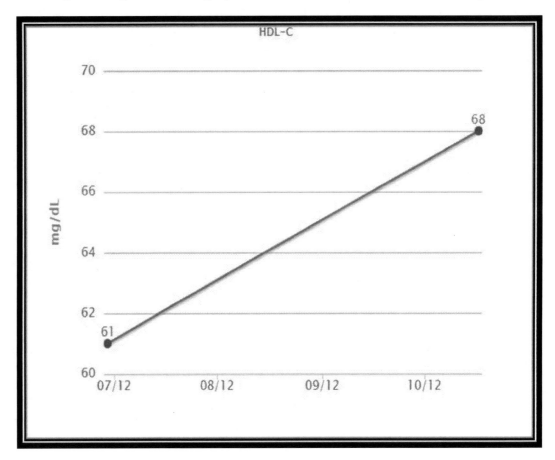

Keep in mind that HDL is the good lipoprotein.

In the graph above, you can see the impact that three months on a low glycemic load diet had on the level of HDL for this 65 year old. This person was also a type 2 diabetic who followed an American Diabetes Association diet for ten years, and had gained an additional 30 pounds for the effort. We will look more closely at the effectiveness of some of the American Diabetes Association guidelines in the upcoming chapter "Receiving the Diagnosis."

In just the first three months of the low glycemic load diet, you can see the HDL level rose seven points. After nine months, forty-five pounds also fell away. These results amazed the physician on the case for over ten years. But do you think this doctor will spread the word about the changes he witnessed? Do you think he will find the time in his busy practice to recommend low glycemic load meal plans to his patients that are now taking statins and metformin to control their conditions?

THIRTY SEVEN TRILLION CELLS

To put heart disease into perspective, let's take a look at the function of the heart, as it relates to our human body. Our heart beats about *one hundred thousand* times each and every single day. During those one hundred thousand beats, our heart sends about two thousand gallons of blood through nearly sixty thousand miles of arteries, capillaries, and veins to deliver freshly oxygenated blood and nutrients to support the approximately thirty seven trillion cells in our human body. These are the amazing works of our circulatory system.

Our bodies are born perfectly designed to carry our being through a long and healthy lifespan. So why are we having so much coronary heart disease among our people? It's not because our hearts are not up to doing their jobs. There's nothing wrong with our hearts. It's not because our arteries, capillaries, and veins forgot how to deliver the freshly oxygenated blood to each of the cells in our bodies. It's not because our cells forgot how to use the fresh supply of blood and the nutrients it contains. And it's not because of "dietary fat", as the mighty Sugar Industry would prefer that we be led to believe.

So what could possibly be threatening this perfectly orchestrated circulatory system? What we are looking for is something independent scientists consider to be scientifically evident, visible, and quantifiable – something able to predict that an event or a set of results will happen again and again, given a set of certain circumstances. We need research that strictly follows the Scientific Method, as we talked about earlier. But what are those scientifically evident, visible and quantifiable circumstances? And just what exactly we are looking for when we are looking for symptoms and results that are definite?

First let's be clear about the fact that there are two types of results, subjective and objective. Any "self-reported" types of symptoms are considered to be *subjective*. Subjective symptoms are those that are reported by individuals as "feeling" states. They may indeed be perceptible, physical, noticeable, real, and quite evident to the person experiencing them. But science has a problem with these types of symptoms, because feeling states are internal and cannot be seen by others from the outside of an individual. That also means that they cannot be accurately and scientifically measured.

Symptoms such as feeling out of breath, dizziness, and tiredness are examples of self-reported subjective symptoms. The information that these types of symptoms give to an individual may indeed be life-changing, but science has no way to measure these sorts of symptoms.

Objective symptoms, on the other hand, are scientific measurements that give us information about the physical state of a person. These can be viewed from outside of the individual. So these objective – scientifically evident, visible, and quantifiable measurements can be used in evaluating the biological processes that are going on inside of an individual.

In the case of heart disease, these objective measurements might include such things as HDL levels, CRP protein (a measure of Inflammation) levels, and blood glucose levels. These objective measurements are also referred to as biomarkers.

Biomarkers are the objective medical measurements that are used in evaluating _biological processes_. Remember the requirements of the scientific method? Results must be reproducible in other subjects given the same set of conditions. Here is what the National Institutes of Health has to say about biomarkers:

"Medical signs have a long history of use in clinical practice—as old as medical practice itself—and biomarkers are merely the most objective, quantifiable medical signs modern laboratory science allows us to measure reproducibly."[19]

So biomarkers are objective, measurable results that are capable of reproduction in other individuals given the same set of conditions.

THEY DREW US A PICTURE

An angel investor, Dr. Arnold van Dyk, of TEMM International (Pty) Ltd funded a special study. A research team in Africa systematically analyzed the data

---

[19] https://www.ncbi.nlm.nih.gov/pmc/articles/PMC3078627/
Accessed 10-10-17

from 294 cohort studies for CHD (coronary heart disease) biomarkers of over a *million* patients. These biomarkers reliably "predict relevant clinical outcomes across a variety of treatments and populations."[20]

The research team dug deep into scientific information hoping to find a graph that would illustrate specific points of data among these 294 studies. They found that no graph existed. Being engineers, they constructed their own graph in order to present the findings of their research. We'll take a look at their first illustrative graph shortly.

The "connection graph" (below) created by these research engineers vividly shows that high glycemic load (HGL) diets go far beyond any commonly associated self-reported (subjective) symptoms.

Their picture includes biomarkers with demonstrated associations of coagulation, inflammation, and vascular function. The researchers include measurable data along with lipid and metabolic symptoms including biomarkers of inflammation, coagulation, and vascular function. You can see the result in the first image, below. You will note that according to these engineers, the greatest contributing factor for Coronary Heart disease is "Food."

---

[20] What are Biomarkers?; Strimbu, K., Tavel, Jorge A. Published in final edited form as: Curr Opin HIV AIDS. 2010 Nov; 5(6): 463–466. https://www.ncbi.nlm.nih.gov/pmc/articles/PMC3078627/ doi: 10.1097/COH.0b013e32833ed177. Accessed 3-27-18.

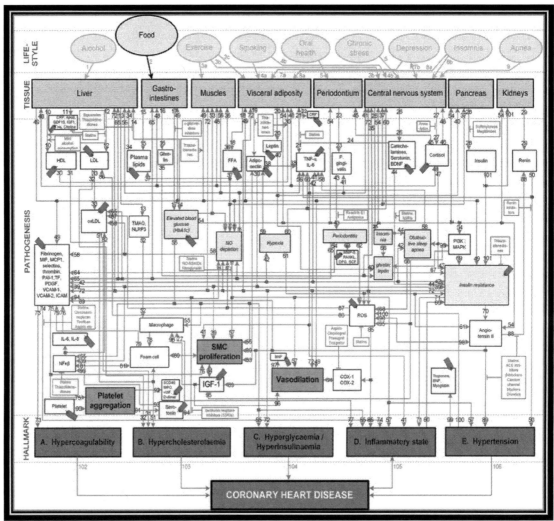

21

In the next graph, you can see that an *increase* LDL (the bad cholesterol) increases the risk for coronary heart disease. And that a *decrease* in HDL levels (the good cholesterol) increases our risk. Many of us are aware of this already.

---

[21] Mathews M, Liebenberg L, Mathews E, et al. ""How do high glycemic load diets influence coronary heart disease?" Nutrition & Metabolism201512:6. DOI: 10.1186/s12986-015-0001-x © Mathews et al.; licensee BioMed Central. March 8, 2015
http://nutritionandmetabolism.biomedcentral.com/articles/10.1186/s12986-015-0001-x
Accessed 11-29-16 at https://nutritionandmetabolism.biomedcentral.com/articles/10.1186/s12986-015-0001-x And https://www.ncbi.nlm.nih.gov/pubmed/25774201
Creative Commons license: https://creativecommons.org/licenses/by/4.0/

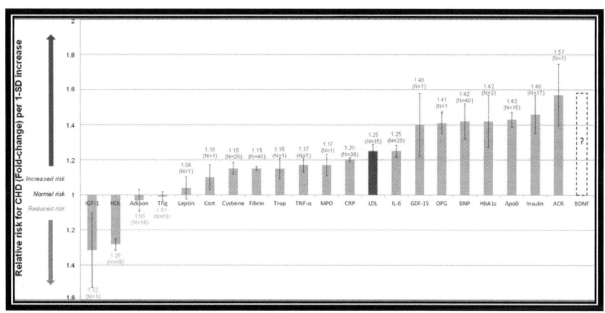

22

The next graph illustrates the effect of high glycemic load diets on other measurable biomarkers as well as HDL and LDL cholesterol levels.

22 Ibid.

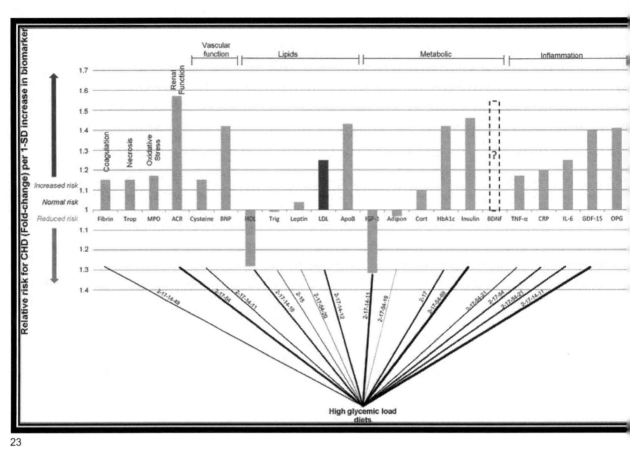

23

DEPRESSION

What is one of the first things we can easily notice when our blood glucose levels fall below where they were even before we ate a high glycemic meal like donuts, pasta or a baked Russet potato?

It may start out subtle, we might begin thinking if only we could eat just a few more bites of that snack we had a little while ago…. Or maybe a few more sips of that soda, just to keep up the energy level we reached right after we ate that last meal. Maybe we have an urge to grab a cup of coffee and a handy candy bar in an effort to prop ourselves back up to how we felt when we had finished eating that high glycemic load meal.

But what if instead, we pause for a moment and listen to the message our body is telling us? We can notice the tiredness, yawning, foggy thinking, feeling cold,

---

[23] Ibid.

and feelings of sadness setting in. This would be a good time to begin journaling your experience.

Dedicate a notebook to this activity. Write down your experience as it unfolds. Begin with what you ate at your most recent meal. List the names and amounts of the foods and beverages you consumed. Write down the date and the time of that meal. Now, write down the date and time when you started noticing tiredness, yawning, foggy thinking, or feeling cold. Write down any feelings of sadness you experience and the time those feelings came to your consciousness. Make a note of how long it took for these feelings to occur after that meal.

Cravings can result as we feel a need to raise our glucose levels, perhaps setting us up for a cycle of binge eating just to keep our blood glucose from falling to such low levels. Keep track of when these cravings occur as well. Feelings of tiredness can lead to distraction, impatience and frustration. These significant symptoms of blood glucose level changes may be reflected in our moods. Feelings of sadness can be confusing for some, and perhaps even disabling for others. Withdrawal from friends and family because of sad moods can cut off the most important support system we have.

These feelings are not imaginary, although they may not be considered scientifically measurable because they are *feeling states*. The image below highlights another kind of actual scientific measurement of what is going on in the situation:

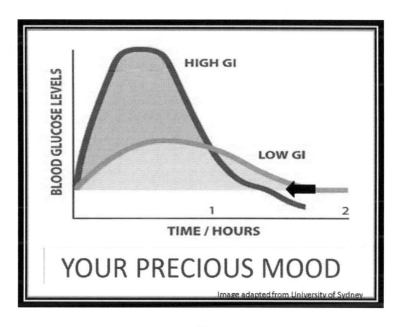

It is real and it is measurable. In the above image, notice the black arrow in the bottom right hand side of the image. Look at the range of blood glucose pointed to by the arrow in that chart for the subject who ate the High GI meal. Notice how blood glucose levels spike when we eat high GI foods and then fall to an even lower level than they were before eating that high GI meal.

It's not just your imagination getting the better of you. And it can certainly affect your thinking and your feelings.

An early eye-opening study by a group of researchers focused on mood and cognition. According to the researchers, the 42 year old volunteers who participated in the study were overweight yet healthy.

Researchers provided all foods, caloric beverages, and a multivitamin supplement to the test subjects for the duration of their six month study. The subjects were randomly assigned to one of two groups: One group received a high glycemic load (HGL) diet; the other received a low glycemic load (LGL) diet.

After the six months of the study, the researchers found the LGL diet to…

"Protect against negative moods which occur during weight loss when a conventional high glycemic diet is consumed."

"Additionally," they explained, "Our results lend support to accumulating evidence of broadly beneficial health effects of low glycemic load diets compared to high glycemic diets in weight management."

And finally, "randomization to the HG diet was associated with a relatively negative change in subclinical depression symptomology over time compared to randomization to the LG diet…and further studies in this area are warranted."[24]

In 2015, a group of psychiatrists at Columbia University Medical Center thought they would do just that. In this study, researchers examined trends in the diet including dietary glycemic index, glycemic load, *types* of carbohydrates

---

[24] Cheatam RA, Roberts S, Das SK, et al. "Long-term effects of provided low and high glycemic load & low energy diet on mood and cognition." *Physiological Behavior*. 2009 September 7:98(3):374-379. DOI: 10.1016/j.physbeh.2009.06.015. Accessed 10-05-16 at: http://www.ncbi.nlm.nih.gov/pmc/articles/PMC2775046/

GLYCEMIC LOAD FOOD GUIDE & PERSONAL WORKBOOK

consumed and other carbohydrate measures (added sugars, total sugars, glucose, sucrose, lactose, fructose, starch, carbohydrate).

A number of experimental studies of small groups with random assignment to high glycemic load diets, even for six month duration had already been found to have negative effects on mood.

A longitudinal epidemiologic study would cover a greater number of people over a longer duration.

The Women's Health Initiative Observational Study (1994-1998) just so happened to recruit just such a cohort. The Columbia University psychiatrists accessed the records of over 70,000 healthy postmenopausal, socioeconomically and racially diverse women from 40 different clinical centers in twenty states.

In the beginning of the Women's Health Initiative, these women completed a 145 item food frequency questionnaire.
Researchers omitted food frequency questionnaires of subjects from this study results if a subject reported having had depression, substance abuse, mental illness, or dementia already.

The psychiatric teams' review supports the association of a high glycemic load diet with depression.

Here is their conclusion:
1. "We found a progressively higher dietary GI to be associated with increasing odds of incident depression.
2. Nonwhole/refined grain consumption was associated with increased odds of depression....
3. The consumption of sweetened beverages, refined foods, and pastries has been shown to be associated with an increased risk of depression.
4. Greater consumption of dietary fiber, whole grains, vegetables and non-juice fruits was associated with decreased risk [for depression]."[25]

The authors caution that the influence of refined carbohydrates on the mood may be in proportion to the amount of refined carbohydrates in the overall diet.

---

[25] Gangwisch J, Hale L, Garcia L, et al." High glycemic index diet as a risk factor for depression: analyses from the Women's Health Initiative." Am J Clin Nutr. 2015 Aug; 102(2):454-63. Doi: 10.3945/ajcn.114.103846. Epub 2015 Jun. Accessed 10-05-16 at: http://ajcn.nutrition.org/content/102/2/454.long#T1

WORLD HEALTH ORGANIZATION PREDICTION

Back in 1996, The World Health Organization predicted that depression would be the second-leading cause of burden on society among all diseases worldwide by the year 2020. [26],[27]

That's this year as of the writing of this book. It is time for us to take notice of this trend. As with any trend, when we look at it without sitting in judgement of it, we can indeed learn something valuable. But we don't have to contribute to it or become part of it.

As evidenced in the following graph, we can see that the average glycemic load (GL) of the diet in the United States rose by a whopping 22% from 1980 to 1990 alone! [28] That's the trajectory we've been on, and we can change course.

---

[26] Ibid.

[27] Murray C, Lopez A. "Evidence-based health policy—lessons from the Global Burden of Disease Study". Science 1996;274:740–3. https://www.ncbi.nlm.nih.gov/pubmed/8966556

[28] Hu F, Stampfer M, Manson J, et al. "Trends in the incidence of coronary heart disease and changes in diet and lifestyle in women." N Engl J Med 2000;343:530–7. Accessed 10-05-16 at: http://www.nejm.org/doi/full/10.1056/NEJM200008243430802#t=article

TABLE 1. AGE-ADJUSTED VALUES FOR DIETARY FACTORS OVER TIME IN THE NURSES' HEALTH STUDY.*

DIETARY FACTOR	1980	1984	1986	1990	P VALUE FOR TREND
Trans fat (% of total energy)	2.20	1.90	1.68	1.52	<0.001
Ratio of polyunsaturated to saturated fat	0.29	0.48	0.47	0.49	<0.001
Cereal fiber (g/day)	2.63	4.21	4.45	4.99	<0.001
Glycemic load†	120.4	138.6	138.0	147.0	<0.001
Marine n−3 fatty acids (% of total energy)	0.05	0.11	0.12	0.14	<0.001
Folate (µg/day)	377	387	403	421	<0.001
Dietary score‡	9.30	13.0	14.0	14.7	<0.001

*Means were standardized according to age distribution for the entire number of person-years of follow-up.

†Glycemic load was calculated by multiplying the carbohydrate content of each food by its glycemic-index value and the frequency of consumption and summing the results for all food items. Each unit of glycemic load represents the equivalent glycemic effect of 1 g of carbohydrate from white bread. Dietary glycemic load represents a diet's overall ability to raise the blood glucose level. [29]

According to the Center for Disease Control, in the U.S. about three quarters of our population is in the grips of a growing obesity and diabetes epidemic. Nearly twenty percent of all of our children and adolescents ages six to nineteen are now considered to be overweight or obese. And if this current obesity trend continues at the same rate as it is now, it could potentially bankrupt our country by 2030 with healthcare costs due to these epidemics alone.

Not only that, but "the global consumption of refined (high glycemic index) foods has also been increasing as regions of the developing world adopt

---

[29] Hu F, Stampfer M, Manson J, et al. "Trends in the incidence of coronary heart disease and changes in diet and lifestyle in women." N Engl J Med 2000;343:530–7. Accessed 10-05-16 at: http://www.nejm.org/doi/full/10.1056/NEJM200008243430802#t=article

western fast-food dietary patterns. There truly is compelling evidence that these two trends are intertwined, and research bears this out."[30]

Over the years, researchers around the world have used methodology established by Drs. Jenkins and Wolever to test the glycemic index and calculate the glycemic load of different foods.

But not all food makers manufacture their creations in different countries, making potential comparisons limited in the first place. "Users should note that manufacturers sometimes give the same product different names in different countries, and in some cases, the same name for different items. Kellogg's Special K and All-Bran, for example, are different formulations in North America, Europe, and Australia."[31] We'll look some specific comparisons in the final chapter of this book.

And not all food makers have been willing to pay for the testing of their products, about $10,000.00 each.

The bottom line on long-term research is found in the 2015 review of The Women's Health Initiative Observational Study on the diets of over 70,000 women. These Columbia University psychiatrists recommend studies that measure overall intakes of carbohydrate and sugar, glycemic index (GI), and glycemic load. So this is no longer just about the obvious obesity and diabetes epidemics. It is just as surely about the perhaps less obvious rate of depression.

The psychiatrists authoring the Columbia University Medical Center study conclude that "randomized trials should be undertaken to examine the question of whether diets rich in low-GI foods could serve as treatments and primary preventive measures for depression."[32]

If you are experiencing sadness, you might keep track of your meals as mentioned earlier. If you find you are eating high GI foods and feeling sad later, you can notice that connection and make adjustments.

---

[30] Gangwisch J, Hale L, Garcia L, et al." High glycemic index diet as a risk factor for depression: analyses from the Women's Health Initiative." Am J Clin Nutr. 2015 Aug;102(2):454-63. Doi: 10.3945/ajcn.114.103846. Epub 2015 Jun Accessed 10-04-16 at: http://ajcn.nutrition.org/content/102/2/454.long

[31] Atkinson FS, Foster-Powell K, Brand-Miller JC. "International tables of Glycemic Index and Glycemic Load Values: 2008." *Diabetes Care*. December; 31(12): 2281-2283. Doi: 10.2337/dc08-1239. Retrieved 9-15-16 from: http://www.ncbi.nlm.nih.gov/pmc/articles/PMC2584181/

[32] Ibid.

HORMONAL RESPONSE

"Refined foods such as white bread, white rice, and soda trigger a hormonal response in the body in order to reduce blood sugar levels. The more *refined* the carbohydrate is, the higher it scores on the glycemic index (GI) scale, and the greater the required hormonal response to reduce the blood sugar levels.

This response may also cause or exacerbate mood changes, fatigue and other symptoms of depression. This suggests that dietary interventions could serve not only as treatments, but also preventive measures for depression." [33]

"The consumption of sweetened beverages, refined foods, and pastries has been shown to be associated with an increased risk of depression in longitudinal studies.

Again, "This response may also cause or exacerbate mood changes, fatigue and other symptoms of depression." [34] However, any influence that refined carbohydrates has on mood could be commensurate with their proportion in the overall diet; studies are therefore needed that [more closely] measure overall intakes of carbohydrate and sugar, glycemic index (GI), and glycemic load." [35]

In 2016, scientists at the Fred Hutchinson Cancer Research Center Division of Public Health Sciences, Seattle, WA, US conducted a *randomized and controlled trial* focusing on the effect of glycemic load and depression.

Considered to be the "gold standard" in clinical trials, a "randomized and controlled trial" serves to isolate a specific variable. In this type of trial, one group receives a particular type of treatment, while another group receives a placebo.

"Eighty-two healthy weight and overweight/obese, but otherwise healthy, adults enrolled in a randomized, crossover controlled feeding study testing low-compared to high-glycemic load diets." [36]

---

[33] Gangwisch J, Hale L, Garcia L, et al." High glycemic index diet as a risk factor for depression: analyses from the Women's Health Initiative." Am J Clin Nutr. 2015 Aug; 102(2):454-63. Doi: 10.3945/ajcn.114.103846. Epub 2015 Jun. Accessed 10-05-16 at: http://ajcn.nutrition.org/content/102/2/454.long#T1

[34] Ibid.

[35] Ibid.

[36] Breymeyer K , Lampe J, McGregor B, Neuhouser M. "Subjective mood and energy levels of healthy weight and overweight/obese healthy adults on high-and low-glycemic load experimental diets." Appetite Science Direct. Volume 107, 1 December 2016, Pages 253–259. Available online 6 August 2016. 2016 Aug 6;107:253-259. doi: 10.1016/j.appet.2016.08.008 Abstract Accessed on 10-04-16 at:

It is important to note two interesting things about this study. None of the subjects had diabetes, and some of the subjects were of healthy weight. So there was no separation of subjects into groups because of weight. The only difference between the two groups was that one group had a *low glycemic load* diet, while the other group had a *high glycemic load* diet.

PROFILE OF MOOD STATES

At the beginning of the study, subjects filled out a questionnaire to evaluate their moods. The "Profile of Mood States" (POMS) instrument was used that includes subscales covering specific psychological dimensions such as:

- anger-hostility,
- confusion-bewilderment,
- depression-dejection,
- fatigue-inertia,
- tension-anxiety,
- vigor-activity,
- total mood disturbance (TMD),
- and negative affect (NA)

"Subjective" mood was evaluated at the beginning and again at the conclusion of the 28-day study feeding periods according to the Center for Epidemiological Studies Depression (CES-D) scale.

All of their diets had the same amount of calories and macronutrient content as a percentage of total energy. The single variable in this study was the *glycemic load* of the two meal plans: One group of subjects had a high glycemic load diet, while the other group had a low glycemic load diet.

The consumption of the high-glycemic load diet resulted in:

- a 38% higher score for depressive symptoms
- 26% higher score for fatigue/inertia
- 55% higher score for Total Mood Disturbance

https://www.ncbi.nlm.nih.gov/pubmed/27507131

- It is also important to note that the overweight/obese participant subgroup had 40% higher scores on the CES-D scale compared to their healthy weight participant counterparts.

The researchers summed up their conclusions this way: "a high-glycemic load diet was associated with higher depression symptoms, total mood disturbance, and fatigue compared to a low-glycemic load diet."[37] While emotions are subjective, that is no biomarkers are evident, they are very real to those who are experiencing them.

They also found this to be especially true (with 40% higher scores) for overweight/obese, but otherwise healthy, adults.

This trial is registered at clinicaltrials.gov: NCT00622661.

[37] Breymeyer K , Lampe J, McGregor B, Neuhouser M. "Subjective mood and energy levels of healthy weight and overweight/obese healthy adults on high-and low-glycemic load experimental diets." Appetite Science Direct. Volume 107, 1 December 2016, Pages 253–259. Available online 6 August 2016. Abstract Accessed 10-04-16 at: https://www.ncbi.nlm.nih.gov/pubmed/27507131

TYPE 2 DIABETES

I f you feel like you might be experiencing any of the less-than-optimal mood symptoms mentioned in the <u>Profile of Mood States survey </u>we just read about, you might just save your life if you look more closely at what is going on with the food in your life. It is possible to recognize how our bodies are responding to different foods as these foods become a part of our bodies through the process of digestion. We just have to pay attention.

ASK YOURSELF THESE QUESTIONS

Here are some things you might consider:
- Do you feel flooded with energy soon after eating some foods?
- Do you feel "jittery," over-energized, or get the "shakes" about half an hour or so after eating some foods?
- Do you feel your energy level begin to fall about three quarter to one hour after you have eaten?
- Are you starting to feel groggy an hour and a half or so after you have eaten a particular food or drink?
- Do you notice feelings of anxiety, frustration, confusion, or sadness two to three hours after eating some foods?
- At about three to four hours after a meal, are you feeling extremely hungry – like you could eat almost anything, and desire something sweet or starchy?
- Do you crave certain foods at the same time every day?
- Are there some foods that you feel you could just eat and eat and never get enough of? Or hurry through eating some foods and yet get the feeling that you never get feeling satisfied?
- Do you start to feel chilly three to four hours after you have eaten some foods?

If you answered yes to any of the questions in the bulleted list above, and you have access to blood glucose testing supplies, you might like to take advantage of the ability to monitor yourself more closely.

You can test before you eat, half an hour later, two hours after, then again at four hours. This will show you how your own body reacts to a specific carbohydrate by providing direct personal feedback. Everybody is somewhat different to some degree in their tolerance and reaction to different carbohydrates. Dedicate a notebook to your results.

Even if you don't use or have access to blood glucose testing supplies, you can still gain valuable feedback by "journaling" your food experiences. Journaling lets you keep track of how you feel half an hour after eating, again at one hour, two hours, three hours, and four hours. This gives you a detailed personalized record of your body's response to different foods. Then you can refer to this record to inspire you while making food choices on a day to day basis.

The reality is that while our mood may often be overlooked, considered as just a minor and subtle symptom to be ignored and overcome, it certainly is important to us personally. In a very real sense, awareness of our mood serves us as an indicator of the "tip of the iceberg." Glycemic Index offers scientific data that can help us recognize the "tip." (We looked at the "association" between Glycemic Index and Depression in the image "Your Precious Mood" in the last chapter on Depression.)

Like the "tip of the iceberg" what is going on under the surface is much greater than what is visible to the eye. And yet if we overlook the subtle "tip," we may not see the iceberg coming.

The fullness of the entire iceberg represents disease states that are measured and diagnosed by physicians and treated by our medical system. But why wait for the entire iceberg to impose itself upon your well-being? Something as delicate as mood is an early warning that we can take advantage of to avoid actual, measurable disease states. We become alert to the potential danger only when we pay attention to our delicate moods.

It may seem strange to think of someone with type 2 diabetes (T2D) as having any kind of advantage, but in a roundabout way, they do. They have a test meter that shows them how their body responds to different foods. A person with T2D is always on the alert to changes in blood sugar levels. The biggest advantage they have is that they measure their blood sugar level many times each day. This is doubly true for someone who is dependent of external insulin.

When they measure their blood sugar level half an hour or one hour after they have eaten a meal containing carbohydrate, they have an opportunity to learn just how much the metabolism of a particular carbohydrate affects their blood sugar level. This information can help them recognize which foods have the least effect on their blood sugar levels and which foods have the greatest effect.

The consequences from lack of care can be dire. But the advantage of self-monitoring is that they don't have to wait for several years to see how it all works out. They don't even have to wait for an annual physical to see how their food choices are affecting their overall health.

By measuring their blood sugar level half an hour after a meal, they get direct results. They know almost right away what happened in their body when they ate that particular food. They know how their body responded right away to that food -- for a fact. That is a fact they can rely on. And it's almost immediate feedback. But it doesn't stop there. When they measure their blood sugar an hour later, and four hours later, they get even more get feedback. All this feedback is powerful information they can use in making the best food choices. They can use this information to reverse T2D, as many people already have. The beauty of numbers, especially personal numbers, is that you can count on them. Numbers do not lie; they always tell you the truth. Numbers can save your life!

As you can see, blood sugar control is not just for the type 2 diabetic. It is also a major factor in heart disease, various cancers, weight control, and a host of other challenges, including our perceived level of happiness.

Reading the scientific research provided in this book puts you in the perfect position to judge the evidence for yourself. Using the Personal Glycemic Load Workbook provided will help you manage your portion sizes so that you can maintain a low glycemic load and naturally control your blood sugar levels.

As we discussed when we viewed the image of what happens when high GI foods are eaten compared to low GI foods – noticing how our body feels can serve as an early warning even for those who do not test their blood sugar levels. This subtle information is something that we can pay attention to long before any disease even begins to take hold, and change our path.

This simple tool can be used by anyone. Even if you don't have access to blood sugar testing supplies you can begin to keep track of how you feel after you eat different foods. And you can even use it before you ever develop any of the kind of symptoms that send you looking for medical care. You'll learn more about how to use it as you read this book.

THE EPIDEMICS

Long before we even had the idea that we were fostering an epidemic of obesity and type 2 diabetes, we learned that we had a growing problem with coronary heart disease (CHD). The startling trend of increasing rates of CHD became obvious in the 1950's. We only recognized that trend when statistics made it obvious. We are going to look closely at that trend to see how and why we, as consumers of modern-day food, were simply blindsided by the entire thing.

Diseases and disorders are merely the byproducts of the way we have lived our lives over many years. Many of the top four diseases and disorders, like heart disease, cancer, depression, and type 2 diabetes hardly existed 75 years ago. But then we weren't consumers of modern-day foods, either.

We all know that as technology has advanced, so has the ability to reach consumers. Consumers are victims of manipulation and corporate greed as never before. Food manufacturers manipulate people in order to make more profits. Just the title, *food manufacturers*, is an <u>oxymoron</u>. We don't manufacture food. Food *grows* with tender loving care. Then we harvest our real food and eat it. Sure, we prepare it in many different ways to create variety in our meals. But the reality is that there is no way to "manufacture" real *food*.

These so-called *food manufacturers* mass produce *food-like products* in order to *profitably* feed a growing population. The only reason they are called food products at all is because the recipes these manufacturers have created do contain SOME remnants of real food. But in many cases there is much less real food in their products than the manufacturers advertising budget leads US to believe....

And these manufacturers create their *food* products in secret ways that will make people crave them. These cravings create an addiction cycle in the consumer. This is very good indeed for their bottom line, because the addiction makes us want to buy more of their products just to feed our addiction. But it has taken us, as a nation of consumers, to an epidemic of seemingly unrelated chronic conditions, such as, you guessed it -- heart disease, cancer, depression, and T2D.

The main perpetrators in this masquerade dress themselves up better than the now popularly suspected common soft drink. They may appear as an "innocent" order of "fries," an aromatic "casserole," or even "100% natural organic fruit juice." And consider this odd-ball fact: Eating a baked Russet potato has an effect on your body that is even *more* powerful than drinking *pure glucose*.

That's right, and many fast food restaurants offer those Russet potatoes as endless side orders in an infinite array of new recipes to tempt your palate. But would you want to drink pure glucose? At least pure glucose is honest about being pure glucose, so you know *in your brain* what your body is dealing with before you lift that glass. But who knows what they have done to those "fries?" And did anyone ever tell you just how damaging a freshly baked Russet potato really is? You'll learn more as you read on.

We can't count on public media to present the truth without bias, because much of their income is derived from their promotions of fast food establishments.

You see, a diagnosis of depression, heart disease, cancer, or type 2 diabetes arrives only after long-time confusion, or a complete lack of information, of how our body responds to certain foods and drinks.

Food manufacturers prosper in the resulting unrestrained insulin response of our bodies that is triggered by their food products. As the peak tapers off, it is followed by unusual feelings of hunger and tiredness, anxiety, sadness, and cravings for more of those foods that we may think we need just to keep us going.

And keep us going, it surely has. But thankfully, now we are armed with over fifty years of data on the subject. That's why we can certainly pinpoint the rising trend in the number of cases of heart disease, cancer, depression, and type 2 diabetes. These top killers flourish because of one main cause.

While type 2 diabetes may not be listed as the number one killer, the main cause of this disease is also at the heart of many other chronic conditions that plague modern humanity. Just some of these health challenges include heart disease, cancer, and depression.

Each of these conditions presents itself in degrees. For instance, type 2 diabetes may begin as insulin resistance, progress to prediabetes, then finally reach the scale of type 2 diabetes. The less dramatic challenges of insulin resistance and prediabetes are really just levels reached along the way to T2D. A diagnosis of insulin resistance is a wake-up call to take action and change the path you are on.

That *Sugar Research Foundation* article mentioned in the beginning of the book quotes a past president of the American Society of Sugar Beet Technology Research as saying that their goal was "to teach people who had never had a course in biochemistry… that sugar is what keeps every human being alive and with <u>energy to face our daily problems</u>." [38] How sad that he saw his life as a set of "daily problems." Perhaps he "practiced what he preached" and ate a lot of sugar, which would explain his lack of energy… .

As a society, we surely have been kept busy dealing with physical disease symptoms caused by long-term high glycemic load lifestyles. What effect does a *symptom treatment lifestyle focus* have on us?

Consider the traffic jams and travel time getting to labs for blood draws, office visits; time spent in waiting rooms, and time and money spent filling prescriptions at pharmacies. Consider the time it takes to understand blood test results and the proper way to use any prescribed medications. Then consider the time spent to earn the money to pay for these things.

Staying occupied with all of this "busyness" takes us further away from the gentle messages our perfectly orchestrated beautiful bodies are constantly sending us. Just getting in touch with ourselves long enough to hear the information our body is giving us could save us a whole lot of time, money, pain, disease, and even an unnecessary early death. Our bodies would be pleased to bless us with the abundance of glowing health and happiness that is our birthright. We just have to allow it. We have to trust our internal wisdom. This is where meditation can play a vital force in our wellbeing.

The first goal of meditation is to become aware of our breathing. This takes our focus away from things outside of ourselves and brings our attention to what our body is doing at this very moment. Meditation calms our mind as well as our body, and puts us in touch with our own inner knowing. We can feel how our body responds to different types of nutrition. But we must pay attention. With wisdom comes knowledge. With knowledge comes responsibility. We must take responsibility for the nourishment that makes us whole. We are more than what we eat, but what we eat can make us more than what we already are.

---

[38] Kearns C., Schmidt L., Glantz S. "Sugar Industry and Coronary Heart Disease Research: A Historical Analysis of Internal Industry Documents." JAMA Intern Med. Published online September 12, 2016. doi:10.1001/jamainternmed.2016.5394 Accessed 10-08-16 at: http://jamanetwork.com/journals/jamainternalmedicine/fullarticle/2548255

Perhaps we have allowed ourselves to be kept too busy to investigate the simple power of using the glycemic index for our mood and our feelings. Glycemic index is not, after all, created to manage mood. But mood is a subtle side effect of how our body responds to variations in dietary glycemic load.

First we have to uncover the fact that there *is* this information available for ourselves in the first place! Then we have to explore the data. While it is by no means complete, there is significant information available for many of the foods in many countries of the world. And there is lots of information on foods in Canada, the United Kingdom, and the USA, plus many other countries, as well.

When we realize that this information about our nutrition exists, we can become knowledgeable about how our bodies respond to different types of food. Studying the information allows us to make more informed food choices. Then we won't be kept as busy with such things as heart disease, cancer, metabolic syndrome, depression, obesity, insulin resistance, and type 2 diabetes.

Aside from what we can learn by reading the scientific results of glycemic index testing, how amazingly wonderful and empowering it is when we realize that our bodies are constantly sending us messages. We have the ability to pay attention to the messages our bodies are telling us. When we recognize how our bodies are responding to different foods, we can break the cycle of disease. And one of the first foods we can minimize is sugar.

Most of our lives are pretty filled with busy schedules. Fast foods are so readily available. Fast food establishments are successful – and continue to pop up all over the place, because they fill the need for fast foods for our fast lives. They are a potential time and perhaps short-term money saver. The trick is being able to create a healthy meal at one of those places. And you'll learn ways to deal with that as you read this book. But first, I'd like to share a personal example.

TONY THE TIGER

I just loved Tony the Tiger when I was a kid. He was so cute, happy, and always full of energy. Tony was my hero. Kellogg's Frosted Flakes were more than breakfast for me. They were a way of life. I believed that if I ate enough of them, I, too, would grow up to be cute, happy, and always full of energy, just like Tony. I ate Frosted Flakes every time I could. I felt certain I could always count on Tony. I was addicted. And I was just lucky that my Mother insisted that I also eat my dinner every day.

I did not know about "marketing" back when I was six years old. But if anyone would have told me that Tony was a marketing gimmick for a cereal manufacturer, I would have shaken my head "no" in disbelief. Tony was my hero, and I believed in him. When I found out what he really was up to, it was like finding out that there really is no Santa Claus.

Kids are likc that, trusting and believing in what they see and hear. That was a long time ago. But the heartache goes on. Not just my own heartache, but the heartache of those whose health suffers, those receiving diagnoses of heart disease, cancer, depression, or type 2 diabetes. And the heartache of those who have lost innocent loved ones to chronic disease. And the worst part of it all is that most of these losses are totally unnecessary. Yet it continues into the twenty first century.

For example, in 2011, Tony's parent, Kellogg's™ created a "Breakfast Council." For their "Breakfast Council" they hired what they called "Independent Dietitians" to promote their products. Here's how it worked: Kellogg's paid these "Independent Dietitian" "Breakfast Council" members to say and do what they wanted them to say and do. Then the "Breakfast Council" members, these "Independent Dietitians" said and did those things. Now, how "independent" is that? One member of the "Council" was even a University Professor. Kellogg's removed their "Breakfast Council" from their website in 2016.

Shame on you, Tony, you are a heartbreaker. We are so totally OVER.

But this really is more like a speck of dust on a crumb. It is easy to mislead children. Children are so trusting and innocent and truthful. Children see no reason to deceive. This kind of stuff has been going on for a long time among chemical, food manufacturing and drug companies. You will understand just how tiny this really is after reading about Project 229, coming up soon.

It is so hard to know who you can trust to tell you the truth, that you really do need to do your own independent research. You deserve to take the time to do this research for your health. You are so worth it. You deserve to do this research for the health of your loved ones. Living a long, healthy life is a privilege you appropriate for yourself and your loved ones by making smart choices. See the results with your own eyes. The health of your human life literally depends on it.

Take this opportunity to empower yourself with scientifically proven methods. Use these methods to cultivate health and happiness for yourself, your family, and other loved ones.

This book would not be complete without with the following information:

- The scientifically proven connection between heart disease, cancer, depression, and type 2 diabetes.
- The secret link between happiness and blood sugar levels that you can use to feel awesome for life.
- Real food examples including prep and serving methods that can be used by anyone to lessen post-prandial glycaemia (high blood sugar).
- A historical timeline of how blood sugar control has evolved over the past century, where we are right now, and how we can create a better future.
- Step-by-step details for using the most revolutionary method of natural blood sugar control.
- Concrete guidance for healing a new diagnosis.
- A Personal Glycemic Load Workbook with step-by-step guidance to let you calculate a low glycemic load for *any* food for successful blood sugar control.

PART 2: THE ADDICTIONS

∽ .... ∾

BRAIN STUDY EVIDENCE

As if food manufacturers had not done enough damage already, there is more. Another problem with foods such as high glycemic carbohydrates is that they automatically fuel sugar addiction.

On June 26, 2013, the American Journal of Clinical Nutrition published a brain imaging study. Scientists used MRI to investigate how the dopamine-containing pleasure centers of the brain might affect food intake.

"Beyond reward and craving, this part of the brain is also linked to substance abuse and dependence, which raises the question as to whether certain foods might be addictive." [39]

This was a randomized, blinded, crossover study, which compared the effects of high and low glycemic meals on two groups of test subjects on two separate days.

After an overnight fast of at least twelve hours, twelve overweight or obese men consumed test meals designed as milkshakes with the same calories, taste and sweetness. One day each subject consumed a high GI milkshake (with quick digesting carbohydrates), on another day, after another overnight fast the same subjects consumed a low GI milkshake (with slow digesting carbohydrates).

"After participants consumed the high-glycemic index milkshake, they experienced an initial surge in blood sugar levels, followed by sharp crash four hours later.

This decrease in blood glucose was associated with excessive hunger and intense activation of the nucleus acumens, a critical brain region involved in addictive behaviors.

Researchers measured blood glucose levels and hunger, while also using functional magnetic resonance imaging (MRI) to observe *brain activity* during

---

[39] Lennerz B, Alsop D, Holsen L., et al. "Effects of dietary glycemic index on brain regions related to reward and craving in men." Adv Nutr July 2015 Adv Nutr vol. 6: 474-486, 2015. doi: 10.3945/?an.115.008268 Full Article Accessed 10-04-16 at: https://www.ncbi.nlm.nih.gov/pmc/articles/PMC3743729/

the crucial four-hour period after a meal, which influences eating behavior at the next meal."[40]

The first innovative aspect of this study is that it is not assessing the effect of calories or sweetness, but the effect of the glycemic index on the glycemic response, measurable in blood glucose levels.

The second innovative aspect of this study is that it uses MRI at four hours, whereas other studies used MRI soon after consumption of the test meals.

This study was designed to compare the effect of high glycemic index carbs (fast digesting) with low glycemic index carbs (slow digesting) four hours after consumption.

TEST MEAL EVIDENCE

Here is a screenshot image depicting the differences in the two milkshake meals. Note the GI for the two meals is located as "Calculated GI" found in the last row, with the High GI milkshake at 84 and the Low GI milkshake at 37:

[40] Boston Children's Hospital. "New brain imaging study provides support for the notion of food addiction." Science Daily. Science Daily, 26 June 2013. Accessed 10-04-16 at: www.sciencedaily.com/releases/2013/06/130626153922.htm.

TABLE 1
Test-meal composition[1]

	High GI	Low GI
Ingredients[2]		
Cornstarch (g)	—	57.2
Light corn syrup (g)	79.0	—
Vanilla extract (g)	7.3	7.3
Milk, 1% fat (g)	—	260.0
Lactaid milk, 1% fat (g)	254.8	—
Egg white, dried (g)	13.0	11.4
Equal[3] (Merisant Co) (g)	2.1	3.1
Olive oil (g)	11.1	10.9
Nutrient composition		
Energy (kcal)	500	500
Carbohydrate (g)	68.9	68.7
Fat (g)	13.7	13.5
Protein (g)	18.1	17.9
Calculated GI[4]	84	37

[1] GI, glycemic index.

[2] Ingredient amounts were scaled so that the meal energy content corresponded to 25% of estimated daily energy requirements. Each participant's high- and low-GI test meals had the same caloric content.

[3] Equal is an artificial sweetener containing aspartame, acesulfame potassium, dextrose, and maltodextrin.

[4] The GI of each meal was calculated by using glucose as a reference standard.

[41]

Keep in mind that up until this point, glycemic index testing lasted for only two hours. This brain imaging study, however, covered four hours in order to determine whether the previous meal would elicit the *"craving" symptom of addiction* at the *next* meal.

Blood samples were drawn before the test began, and every half hour over the four hour test period.

---

[41] Lennerz B, Alsop D, Holsen L., et al. "Effects of dietary glycemic index on brain regions related to reward and craving in men." Adv Nutr July 2015 Adv Nutr vol. 6: 474-486, 2015. doi: 10.3945/?an.115.008268 Full Article Accessed 10-04-16 at: https://www.ncbi.nlm.nih.gov/pmc/articles/PMC3743729/

INSULIN RESPONSE EVIDENCE

Below is a screenshot of how the blood sugar (blood glucose) and insulin levels of the subjects responded during this four hour test experience:

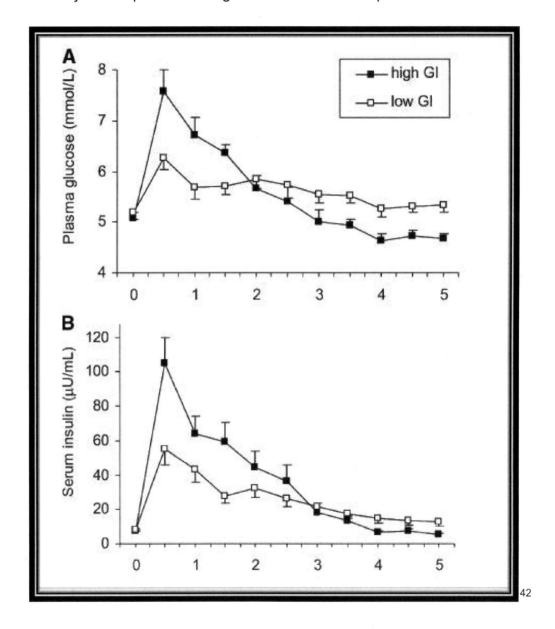

This is what the scientists have to say about their groundbreaking four hour testing experience:

[42] Lennerz B, Alsop D, Holsen L., et al. "Effects of dietary glycemic index on brain regions related to reward and craving in men." Adv Nutr July 2015 Adv Nutr vol. 6: 474-486, 2015. doi: 10.3945/?an.115.008268 Full Article Accessed 10-04-16 at: https://www.ncbi.nlm.nih.gov/pmc/articles/PMC3743729/

"The decrease in blood glucose, which often falls below fasting concentrations by 4 h after a high-GI meal, may lead to excessive hunger, overeating, and a *preference* for foods that *rapidly restore blood glucose to normal* (i.e. high GI), propagating cycles of overeating.

Compared with an isocaloric low-GI meal, a high-GI meal decreased plasma glucose, increased hunger, and selectively stimulated brain regions associated with reward and craving in the late postprandial period, which is a time of special significance to eating behavior at the next meal.

These neurophysiologic findings, together with longer feeding studies of weight-loss maintenance suggest that *reduced consumption of high-GI carbohydrates* (specifically, highly processed grain products, potatoes, and concentrated sugar) may ameliorate overeating and facilitate maintenance of a healthy weight in overweight and obese individuals." [43]

ADVERTISING EVIDENCE

To compound the existing problem is the current culture of advertising. Many triggers for high glycemic load foods are ever-present on billboards, television commercials, and in social and other media of every kind.

"Human brain studies show that mesolimbic dopamine pathways activated in response to palatable foods are the same as those activated in drug addiction and can trigger withdrawal effects similar to those seen with *opioid* drugs.

These reward pathways can be triggered by environmental cues that indicate the availability of food."[44] "They can motivate consumption even in the absence of hunger and bias choices toward them. Advertising fosters associations between these cues and activities such as sport and socializing, and the relation between branding and advertising and food intake has been demonstrated."[45], [46]

---

[43] Lennerz B, Alsop D, Holsen L., et al. "Effects of dietary glycemic index on brain regions related to reward and craving in men." Adv Nutr July 2015 Adv Nutr vol. 6: 474-486, 2015. doi: 10.3945/?an.115.008268 Full Article Accessed 10-04-16 at: https://www.ncbi.nlm.nih.gov/pmc/articles/PMC3743729/

[44] Johnson F, Wardle J, "Variety, Palatability, and Obesity."Adv Nutr November 2014 Adv Nutr vol. 5: 851-859, 2014 doi: 10.3945/an.114.007120. Accessed 10-07-16 at: http://advances.nutrition.org/content/5/6/851.full#xref-ref-125-1

The fact is that we regularly face many "food prompt" triggers designed by highly skilled, highly paid professionals planned to affect our choices in food selection.

For example, at a movie theatre, there may be subliminal frames inserted into the movie depicting soda, candy bars, or other things available at the refreshment stand. Bringing your own bag of nuts or other low glycemic snacks is an option.

[45] Ziauddeen H, Alonso M, Hill James, J., et al. "Obesity and the Neurocognitive Basis of Food Reward and the Control of Intake." Adv Nutr July 2015 Adv Nutr vol. 6: 474-486, 2015. Doi: 10.3945/an.115.008268. Accessed 10-07-16 at: http://advances.nutrition.org/content/6/4/474.full

[46] Burger S, Stice E. "Neural responsivity during soft drink intake, anticipation, and advertisement exposure in habitually consuming youth." Obesity (Silver Spring) 2014; 22:441–50. 174. Full Article Accessed 10-07-16 at: https://www.ncbi.nlm.nih.gov/pmc/articles/PMC4005612/

CONFLICTS OF INTEREST

At that time "*Dietary Fats, Carbohydrates and Atherosclerotic Disease*," (the Hegstead, McGandy, and Stare) research review was published in the *New England Journal of Medicine* in 1967, it actually was unnecessary to list any possible conflicts of interest on scientific papers. That's one reason the *Sugar Research Foundation* got away with their deceit.

The conflict of interest requirement didn't begin until the 1980's, which gave the sugar industry more than a twenty year lead.

And by the 1980's, no one even suspected the role sucrose played in CHD. By this time sucrose (sugar) became an addictive additive incorporated into so many consumables, it became difficult to find a manufactured food product without added sugar!

It was also in 1980 that the US adopted its first set of dietary guidelines. The US developed these guidelines to advise consumers on how to avoid the ever-increasing risk of CHD. The dietary guidelines recommended a lower daily allowance of fat, saturated fat, and cholesterol. This conveniently left a void of about twenty percent of daily caloric intake. How profitable for the sugar industry -- creating such a void -- to be filled with carbohydrates such as added sugar (sucrose).

And all of this happened because of such highly respected and distinguished scientists.

Was their work criminal? Yes. Theirs was a moral crime against all of humanity. They sold us out, broke our trust, and killed our loved ones. They caused needless pain and suffering. Their advice gave many of us potentially fatal diseases. Then as other countries adopted western lifestyles, our brothers and sisters in these countries suffered the same fate.

But it took over fifty years to even begin to find out. And the scoundrels who perpetrated this scam have already died. I wonder if any of them choked to death on a mouth full of table sugar or maybe even Sugar Frosted Flakes....

The only way we can know the truth about our food is to do our own research. We need to see research done by independent scientists, rather than research "sponsored" by corporations to promote their products. And then it is up to us as individuals to share the information we find with others as best we can.

THE SWEET DECEPTION

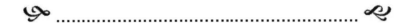

As the rates of coronary heart disease began a noticeable rise during the 1950's, researchers began compiling statistics in hopes of locating some commonality among its victims.

Then, in June, 1965, the *Annals of Internal Medicine* published "Carbohydrates and Cholesterol Metabolism"[47] linking sucrose (table sugar) to coronary heart disease (CHD.) The first two articles covered reports of an epidemiological study suggesting that blood glucose levels were a better predictor of atherosclerosis than either serum cholesterol levels or hypertension. The third article demonstrated that sucrose, more than starches, aggravated carbohydrate-induced hypertriglyceridemia and hypothesized that "perhaps fructose, a constituent of sucrose but not of starch, [was] the agent mainly responsible."[48]

An accompanying editorial argued that these findings corroborated John Yudkin's research (his book, *Pure, White, and Deadly* was finally published in 1972). Yudkin maintained that if elevated serum triglyceride levels were a CHD risk factor, then "sucrose (a combination of glucose and fructose) must be atherogenic." [49]

On July 11, 1965, the New York Tribune ran an article explaining that, while sugar's association with atherosclerosis was proven only by limited studies, this new research fortified the case that sugar increased the risk of heart attacks.

---

[47] Ibid.

[48] Kearns C., Schmidt L., Glantz S. "Sugar Industry and Coronary Heart Disease Research: A Historical Analysis of Internal Industry Documents." JAMA Intern Med. Published online September 12, 2016. doi:10.1001/jamainternmed.2016.5394 Accessed 10-08-16 at:
http://jamanetwork.com/journals/jamainternalmedicine/fullarticle/2548255

[49] Kearns C., Schmidt L., Glantz S. "Sugar Industry and Coronary Heart Disease Research: A Historical Analysis of Internal Industry Documents." JAMA Intern Med. Published online September 12, 2016. doi:10.1001/jamainternmed.2016.5394 Accessed 10-08-16 at:
http://jamanetwork.com/journals/jamainternalmedicine/fullarticle/2548255

PROJECT 229

Two days after the New York Tribune article hit the newsstands, on July 13, 1965, the *Sugar Research Foundation* (SRF) created and funded Project 229 in order to take the heat off of sucrose. Project 229 would be a published research review on the problems created by dietary fat and cholesterol, to make sugar appear to be an innocent bystander despite earlier epidemiologic studies showing that in fact, sucrose consumption was a major risk factor in CHD that had begun sweeping our nation.

Frederick Stare served as Chair of Harvard's School Public Health and Nutrition Department. He and two of his staff signed on to create "a review article of the several papers which find some special metabolic peril in sucrose and, in particular, fructose,"[50] and to see to it that their review article was published.

D. Mark Hegsted, Robert McGandy, and Frederick Stare wrote the review, "Dietary Fats, Carbohydrates and Atherosclerotic Disease." Their review was published in the New England Journal of Medicine (NEJM) in two parts in 1967. They were prominent Harvard University Professors (who accepted about $25,000.00 down and another $25,000.00 upon publication (in 2016 dollars).

These professors criticized evidence from randomized human clinical trials, epidemiologic studies, and mechanistic studies showing sucrose consumption to be a high risk factor for CHD. The review downplayed evidence that sucrose was the problem and pointed to dietary fat and cholesterol as the culprit.

They [further] argued that the "lack of mechanistic evidence confirming the biological plausibility that dietary cholesterol and saturated fat raised serum cholesterol levels was unimportant."[51]

The authors of this research review claimed that they received funding from the "Nutrition Foundation," while they avoided mentioning the funding that they received from the sugar associations' Washington lobbying branch, the *Sugar Research Foundation* (SRF). Without owning up to SRF sponsorship, the research reviews deliberately and effectively turned the view of the scientific community away from results of then-current epidemiological and

---

[50] Ibid.
[51] Kearns C., Schmidt L., Glantz S. "Sugar Industry and Coronary Heart Disease Research: A Historical Analysis of Internal Industry Documents." JAMA Intern Med. Published online September 12, 2016. doi:10.1001/jamainternmed.2016.5394 Accessed 10-08-16 at: http://jamanetwork.com/journals/jamainternalmedicine/fullarticle/2548255

other scientific study reviews that stressed the association of sugar consumption (sucrose) as the most highly probable instigator of heart disease.

In this "bought by the sugar industry" review, the "paid-off" scientists reported that there was evidence that dietary cholesterol and saturated fat are what really caused the increasing statistics of heart disease. They argued that the best approach to avoid heart disease was to reduce dietary cholesterol and substitute polyunsaturated fat for saturated fat in the diet, which should be easy, since it was plentifully available. The scientists took the stand of:

- Never mind that most current scientific studies show that sucrose consumption is strongly linked to heart disease.
- Never mind that the fifty percent of fructose that makes up sucrose (sugar) appears to be a major factor according to scientific research results.
- Never mind the complete lack of evidence showing that dietary cholesterol and saturated fat could even possibly raise serum cholesterol levels.
- And they totally omitted the fact that blood glucose levels are a better predictor of atherosclerosis than serum cholesterol levels or even hypertension.

And on that stand they formulated their "review" of the current scientific studies to make adding sugar to our food supply seem like a really smart idea. This in turn would serve to increase the consumption of sugar in the diet by at least 20 percent. They were quite successful.

Their review concluded that there was "no doubt" that the only dietary intervention required to prevent CHD was to reduce dietary cholesterol and substitute polyunsaturated fat for saturated fat in the American diet."[52]

Stare was an expert in dietary causes of CHD and had been consulted by many august bodies including the National Heart Institute, and American Heart Association, as well as by food companies and trade groups. No wonder this report seemed credible and everyone fell for it. Over fifty years passed as we helplessly witnessed rising rates in CHD and other seemingly unrelated noncommunicable diseases such as cancer, depression and type 2 diabetes. That is, until some Health Policy Study researchers made a discovery -- that is not publicized in mainstream media.

A SPECIAL COMMUNICATION

---

[52] Ibid.

In 2016, at the Philip R. Lee Institute for Health Policy Studies, San Francisco, California, Cristin Kearns, Laura Schmidt, and Stanton Glantz created a timeline using *internal sugar industry documents* beginning as early as the 1950's.

These Health Policy Study researchers located and combed through 346 documents, totaling 1582 pages to create their timeline: *"Sugar Industry and Coronary Heart Disease Research: A Historical Analysis of Internal Industry Documents."*

Their research finally blew the lid off the commonly recommended low-fat diet that has been promoted since the 1980's to combat the growing ranks of heart disease.

The Special Communication, published by the Journal of the American Medical Association on September 12, 2016, details the communication chain outlining the successful efforts of the sugar industry to influence public health policy and the scientific debate regarding sugar and CHD.

About a month later, on Saturday, October 8, 2016 at 5:30 a.m. EST, live on CNBC, Breaking News Anchor Sue Herera interviewed Cristin Kearns (author of the 2016 JAMA Special Communication) and the current President and CEO of the Sugar Association, Courtney Gaine. You can see the video of the interview at this link to CNBC article or by following the link in the footnotes below for more on the subject. [53]

You can also review the "Special Communication of The American Medical Association," available link to AMA Special Communication or by following the link in the footnotes below. [54]

This Special Communication comes more than fifty years after the fact. Fifty years which saw dramatic changes in public health dietary recommendations that were supposed to help us all avoid CHD.

You may have already heard of this Special Communication if you are a member of the Journal of the American Medical Association. But maybe you are not a member. As a professional, the Journal of the American Medical

---

[53] http://www.cnbc.com/2016/10/07/sugar-vs-fat-debate-gets-new-life-after-study-casts-doubt-on-consensus.html

[54] Kearns C., Schmidt L., Glantz S. "Sugar Industry and Coronary Heart Disease Research: A Historical Analysis of Internal Industry Documents." JAMA Intern Med. Published online September 12, 2016. doi:10.1001/jamainternmed.2016.5394 Accessed 10-08-16 at: http://jamanetwork.com/journals/jamainternalmedicine/fullarticle/2548255

Association will allow you to purchase the right to read the full <u>article here</u>[55] for 24 hours for $30.00.

Obviously, this article is intended for members of the Journal of American Medical Association, and not really meant for public consumption. I wonder how long it will take for this information to be available to the public. I think we all deserve to know the truth right now. I think we have lost enough of our health and loved ones to chronic diseases already. Why wait for the information to trickle down to the rest of us? Who knows if or when that will ever happen, unless you and I take action?

The only reason I learned about this Special Communication is because of Sue Herera. Her story aired live at 5:30 a.m. on a Saturday morning. I found the story in my news feed at about 7:00 am. Now how many of us are watching the news at 5:30 a.m. on a Saturday morning after working all week long? By Sunday, the article was no longer in the newsfeed. That was such a small window for such vitally important information.

Who would have thought that it would take us fifty years to discover such a deadly global fraud? The truth is finally available, even if only to subscribers of the Journal of the American Medical Association.

But how long will it take until our doctors, members of the Journal of the American Medical Association, read it? How many of these member doctors will research the information in the article and review the scientific studies presented?

How many of these member doctors can afford to take the time to apply what they learn to their already busy practice? How many of these member doctors will share the information they learn with their patients? And let's take this a step further: How many of these physicians will continue to research until they discover what happens to our bodies when we metabolize other carbohydrate foods that quickly turn into sugar during the process of digestion? What about that? Will we ever get there on a global scale? How long should we wait for this information to become mainstream? Or will we be much better off if we do our own research?

---

[55] http://jamanetwork.com/journals/jamainternalmedicine/fullarticle/2548255

SWEET LITTLE LIES

We can understand why it is *not* in the best financial interest of food and beverage manufacturers to remove added sugars (sucrose) from their food-like products. After all, sucrose is just a really inexpensive combination of glucose and fructose.

In an "Invited Commentary," Marion Nestle, Dept. of Nutrition and Food Studies at New York University delivered a response to the article written by Kearns, published by JAMA. In the Invited Commentary titled "Food Industry Funding of Nutrition Research: The Relevance of History for Current Debates," Nestle poses the question, "Is it really true that food companies deliberately set out to manipulate research in their favor? And she answers that question with, "Yes. It is, and the practice continues."[56]

"The documents leave little doubt that the intent of the industry-funded review was to reach a foregone conclusion..." It's not just historical either. Nestle goes on to say, "In 2015, the New York Times obtained emails revealing Coca-Cola's cozy relationship with sponsored researchers who were conducting studies aimed at minimizing the effects of sugary drinks on obesity."[57] But the reality is that the effects of sugary drinks and quickly digested carbohydrates are not minimized at all, the only thing minimized is the *public's awareness* of the negative effects....

---

[56] Nestle, Marion. "Food Industry Funding of Nutrition Research: The Relevance of History for Current Debates." JAMA Internal Medicine 176.11 (2016): 1685-1686.
[57] Ibid.

UNDERSTANDING CARBOHYDRATE METABOLISM: A TIMELINE

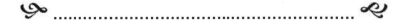

S cientists have long been searching for ways to understand and control the sugar levels in our blood. Earlier in the twentieth century, young children usually died from the disease of diabetes at an early age.

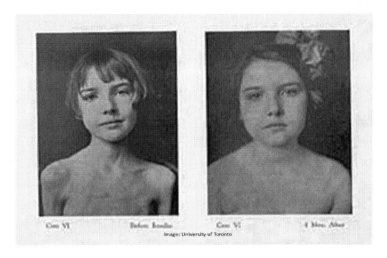

Image: University of Toronto

You can see the results of the early treatment in the above, left photo. The only known "remedy" in the early 1900's to postpone death from diabetes was <u>a starvation diet</u>. Eating only 400-600 calories a day would extend their expected lifespan to 4-5 years. Without this type of intervention, a child with a diabetes diagnosis would only live for 12 to 18 months.

Children received opium to make them less aware of the pain they suffered, and the abominable "<u>Allen Diet</u>" was followed. This diet starved patients until their urine contained no sugar, then the diet gradually reintroduced more food until the number of calories to maintain a sugarless state was established.

In the above image on the right, you can see the same girl after treatment with <u>insulin</u>. She was one of the fortunate few who survived the only treatment that was available at the time. Lucky for her, researchers came up with a solution that saved her life.

Frederick Banting (1891-1941) was born in Ontario, Canada. As a young boy, he watched as a childhood friend of his died of <u>diabetes</u> at the age of twelve.

As a young man, in the spring of 1921, <u>Dr. Frederick Banting</u> moved into a seven by nine foot flat at the University of Toronto. He had no more than an idea, and he set about his research to discover an alternative to starvation for blood sugar control.

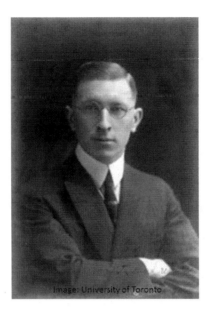

His idea was that a certain part of the <u>pancreas</u> produced a substance capable of treating diabetes. Banting and his colleague, Charles Best, started by using dogs for their test experiments. But they needed the financial backing in the form of a sponsorship and they needed a laboratory.

<u>John James Richard Macleod</u> was professor of physiology at the University of Toronto. He was also one of the most prominent experts on <u>carbohydrate metabolism</u> at that time. As Macleod was taking a summer vacation, he offered the use of a laboratory to Banting for his research. It was there that Banting and Best began the work of isolating the crucial substance that would one day be recognized as the agent responsible for carbohydrate metabolism.

In less than two years, Banting and Best made the great discovery of insulin. In 1923, Banting and his colleagues received the Nobel Prize for their efforts.

Through their research, they learned that insulin was universal among differing species. In fact, they discovered that the insulin produced by dogs and cattle was not only safe, but effective for human use. They were breaking ground on a new life-saving discovery. They needed human test subjects for this newly isolated substance. Rather than risk harming others, they tested the substance on *themselves.*

The success of Banting's team of researchers brought an overwhelming demand for this newly discovered effective blood sugar regulation substance. The need was so great in fact that the production of this miracle drug was turned over to Ely Lilly and Company to keep up with the growing demand for their product.

To date, Banting's discovery has saved over eighteen billion lives.[58]

---

[58] Breecher MM, Anderson T. "Frederick Banting MD." *ScienceHeroes.com*. Retrieved 10-10-17 from: http://scienceheroes.com/index.php?option=com_content&view=article&id=80&Itemid=115

INTRODUCING THE GLYCEMIC INDEX

✑ .... ✑

Sixty years after Banting and Best discovered insulin at the University of Toronto in 1981, Dr. David Jenkins and Dr. Thomas Wolever proposed the concept of a glycemic index for all carbohydrate containing foods. The index measures how the blood sugar levels in our bodies respond to the various "personalities" of different carbohydrate foods.

Their studies included eight to ten volunteers. After an overnight fast, these volunteers ate individual foods in amounts that contained 50g. of carbohydrate. (Note: The *volume* or *weight* of the food or drink did not matter. The only requirement was that a serving contain 50 g. of carbohydrate.) After consuming the test food (or drink), blood glucose was measured and recorded at fifteen minute intervals for two hours.

As a control, these same subjects returned at a later date, again after an overnight fast. This time they drank a 50 g. carbohydrate portion of pure glucose (with a glycemic index of 100.) Again blood glucose levels were measured and recorded at fifteen minute intervals for two hours.

The *American Journal of Clinical Nutrition* published the results of Jenkins and Wolevers' initial 62 different food test results: *"Glycemic index of foods: a physiological basis for carbohydrate exchange."* in 1981. [59]

The glycemic index mainly ranges from 0 to 100+. Foods rank on the glycemic index according to their potential to raise blood sugar levels as compared to glucose raising blood sugar at 100%. That means a glycemic index of 50 raises blood sugar levels only 50% as high as does pure glucose.

The glycemic index researchers saw a noticeable trend among 50g carbohydrate servings of *high* glycemic vs *low* glycemic foods, and plotted the results of their two hour testing results on a graph for comparison. On the graph below, you can clearly see the different effects of high GI foods (shown in red)

---

[59] Jenkins D, Wolever T, Taylor R, et al. "Glycemic index of foods: a physiological basis for carbohydrate exchange." *American Journal of Clinical Nutrition.* 1981. March; 34(3):362-366. Retrieved from: https://academic.oup.com/ajcn/article-abstract/34/3/362/4692881?redirectedFrom=fulltext

on blood glucose levels compared to the effects of low GI foods (shown in yellow) on blood glucose levels.

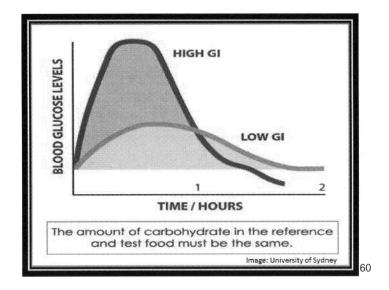

You will notice in the above image that *high GI* foods raise blood glucose levels quickly. Blood glucose reaches a peak in about half an hour. After that peak, blood glucose levels begin to fall quite rapidly. You may also notice that in the case of the *high GI* food, the level continues to fall to a level that is even *lower than before eating the high GI food* beginning at about an hour and forty five minutes. This will become quite significant later when we look more closely at how our bodies respond when this happens.

In contrast, the blood glucose level rises gently after eating a *low GI* food. In about half an hour, it begins a mild gradual descent and finally comes to rest at the point where it was before the meal. The significance of this divergence will become even more significant later, when we consider some more subtle issues, like how blood glucose levels affect hunger, cravings, and our precious mood.

Consider for a moment the effects of two foods, broccoli and glucose. In the image below, notice how much broccoli a subject would have to consume in order to consume 50 g. of carbohydrate of broccoli compared to 50 g. of glucose:

---

[60] www.glycemicindex.com

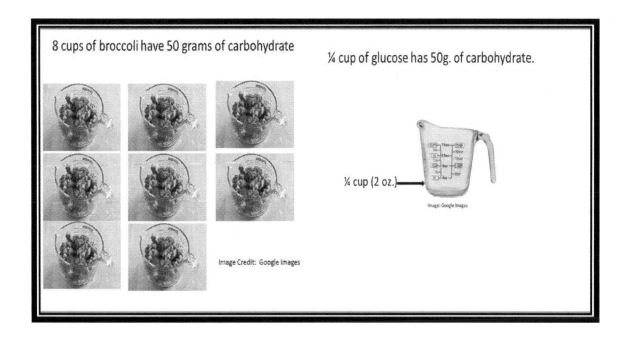

While it takes only 59 mL (or 2 oz.) of glucose to deliver 50g of carbohydrate, it takes 1,896 mL (or 8 cups) of chopped broccoli to deliver 50g of carbohydrate. (This is one key to why most leafy vegetables are so good for blood sugar control. Another key is the amount of fiber they contain.)

Now which of the two would fill you up faster and keep you full longer? Some foods, like broccoli, are not even listed among the glycemic index entries. These foods have been "assigned" a glycemic value because no one can eat 1896 mL (or 8 cups) of broccoli at a sitting. We will go deeper into the details of these types of foods later.

The following simple chart gives you an idea of what it means to have a low, medium, and high glycemic index food. But you must be cautioned that there is a broad range in the placement of these glycemic index rankings. For instance, to be considered "medium" glycemic, the range is from 56 to 69. That is a difference of 13 points. This difference is actually quite significant when we calculate glycemic load. And we will cover this subject thoroughly throughout the rest of this book.

> Glycemic Index:
> Low: 0 – 55
> Medium: 56 – 69
> High: 70+

IS AN INSULIN INDEX MORE ACCURATE?

Not to leave any stone unturned, researchers in the department of biochemistry, at the University Sydney were also testing and charting the effects of carbohydrate foods. In 1995, the American Journal of Clinical Nutrition published the "*International tables of glycemic index*" by Kay Foster-Powel and Jennie Brand Miller. By this time the glycemic index testing results grew tenfold to include nearly 600 foods.[61]

In 1997, Foster-Powel and Brand-Miller wondered if there might be a better way to anticipate blood sugar levels. These scientists proposed that an "Insulin Index" might prove to be a more accurate a gauge of insulin response.

To study their theory, they tested thirty eight foods much in the same way as testing for glycemic index. After an overnight fast, eleven to thirteen healthy adults ate prescribed amounts of test foods. They recorded blood glucose levels of the volunteers every fifteen minutes over a two hour period. One difference in the testing process was that they used white bread (given a value of 100%) instead of glucose as the reference food. Another difference was that they measured the amount of the test food in *calories* rather than in *carbohydrate* content.

These researchers reported that "overall, glucose and insulin scores were highly correlated. However, protein-rich foods and bakery products (high in fat and refined carbohydrate) elicited "insulin" responses that were disproportionately higher than their "glycemic" responses." [62]

---

[61] Foster-Powel K, Miller JB. "International tables of glycemic index. " *American Journal of Clinical Nutrition*. 1995. October; 62(4):8715-8905. Retrieved from: http://ajcn.nutrition.org/content/62/4/871S.abstract

[62] Holt H, Miller J, Petocz P. "An insulin index of foods: the insulin demand generated by 1000-kJ portions of common foods". Am J Clin Nutr November 1997

They also reported that the test results compiled for the 38 foods tested for their "insulin index" had a high level of uncertainty.

Another important factor unaccounted for in this study is the effect of gluconeogenesis[63]. This natural metabolic process turns non-carbohydrates such as protein and fat into glucose. The effect of gluconeogenesis is particularly evident in the *second* hour of the two hour blood glucose level readings recorded by researchers. And it is also one of the reasons that the ketogenic diet may help people lose weight.

WHO AND FAO

Recognizing the mounting evidence of the human glycemic response on health, in 1997 the Food and Agriculture Organization (FAO) of the United Nations and the World Health Organization (WHO) organized a committee of experts to review the research evidence regarding carbohydrates in human nutrition and health. The committee "endorsed the use of the Glycemic Index (GI) method for classifying carbohydrate rich foods *and recommended that the GI values of foods be used in conjunction with information about food composition to guide food choices.*"[64]

That would seem to mean that they recommend that the GI values be available with the rest of the nutrition information about a food. Wouldn't a convenient location for this information be on the label of each manufacturer prepared food? And how about including this information in the country's USDA National Nutrient Database files, Food Data Central? Display of this crucial data would provide another opportunity for the consumer to take charge of their health and well-being. And these small pieces of information would make it much easier for the consumer to easily calculate the glycemic load. Or better yet, the files would update to display the glycemic load of a food depending upon the serving size selected. That is how this Personal Glycemic Load Food Guide & Personal Workbook is set up.

---

vol. 66 no. 5 1264-1276
Accessed: October 2, 2016 at: http://ajcn.nutrition.org/content/66/5/1264.abstract
[63] https://en.wikipedia.org/wiki/Gluconeogenesis
[64] Foster-Powell K, Holt S, Brand-Miller J.
"International table of glycemic index and glycemic load values: 2002."
Am J Clin Nutr January 2002 vol. 76 no. 1 5-56
Retrieved from: http://ajcn.nutrition.org/content/76/1/5.full

If we would have listened to the recommendations of the Food and Agriculture Organization (FAO) of the United Nations and the World Health Organization back in 1997 -- to include the GI ranking with the rest of our food composition information, this book would likely not be needed.

THE GLYCEMIC LOAD

It was also in 1997 that Harvard University professors led by Dr. Walter Willet introduced the concept of the glycemic load. This is a single number that takes into account not only the glycemic index but also the total number of grams of available carbohydrate in a serving. The glycemic load is a simple calculation that arrives at a single number based on the carbohydrate content and the glycemic index of a food. Glycemic load is the *comprehensive* measure of the glycemic response. In order to calculate the glycemic load, the glycemic index is a necessity, and the amount of available carbohydrate in a serving is required.

Here is a simple chart on glycemic load scores:

> Glycemic Load:
> Low: 0 – 10
> Medium: 11 – 19
> High: 20 +

By 2002, researchers had collected and organized the test results of 1300 foods. The American Journal of Clinical Nutrition published this record as the *"The International Tables of Glycemic Index and Glycemic Load Values: 2002."* [65] At this time, both the *glycemic index* and the *glycemic load* of these 1300 foods became available in the tables.

Here is what the authors of this collection said: "The GI has proven to be a more useful nutritional concept than is the chemical classification of

[65] ibid

carbohydrate (as simple or complex, as sugars or starches, or as available or unavailable) permitting new insights into the important relation between the physiologic effects of carbohydrate-rich foods and health." [66]

In 2002, the University of Sydney began to publish the results of these tests on their website at http://www.glycemicindex.com/. You can search for different foods on this website and see how they score. Be sure to verify that you look at results based on foods in your own country, as well as review the details of the test results. There are some significant differences based on the country a food is produced in. Being an online resource makes it easily adapted for updating the collection with new test results as they become available.

The most recent compilation of GI/GL information is published by Diabetes Care and archived by the U.S. National Institutes of Health. *"The International Tables of Glycemic Index and Glycemic Load Values: 2008"* contain nearly *three thousand* food test results on human subjects.[67] The results are available for your review free of charge. You can click on the link or access through the footnote below. This excellent resource contains several *"Supplemental"* Tables and is now accessible for online viewing only. For many years it was also downloadable to a computer desktop and accessible to the user even without being online.

I promised to get back to discuss publications marked as "supplements" later. Now is the time. When we looked at the antics of Kellogg's earlier, we learned that they marked some of their materials as "Supplements." We also see that the 2008 International Tables (above) are also available as Supplemental Tables. Supplement means addition, complement, add-on, insert. And according to the Journal of the Academy of Nutrition and Dietetics, editorial standards for supplements are the same as for regular articles.[68] So there is only room to tell the truth to consumers of these products to have an article published here.

"Supplements" are also referred to as *advertising.* That's because specific manufacturers of specific products are listed. You will notice that *The International Tables of Glycemic Index and Glycemic Load Values: 2008* contains "Supplemental Tables." These "Supplements" include the tables that

---

[66] Powel K, Holt, S, Miller J. "International table of glycemic index and glycemic load values: 2002." *American Journal of Clinical Nutrition.* 2002. January; 76(1):5-56. Retrieved from: http://ajcn.nutrition.org/content/76/1/5.full

[67] Atkinson F, Foster-Powell K, Brand-Miller J."International tables of Glycemic Index and Glycemic Load Values: 2008." *Diabetes Care.* December; 31(12): 2281-2283. Doi: 10.2337/dc08-1239. Retrieved from: http://www.ncbi.nlm.nih.gov/pmc/articles/PMC2584181/

[68] http://www.cnbc.com/2016/11/21/how-kellogg-paid-independent-experts-to-tout-cereal.html Accessed 11-25-16

list the GI/GL values of individual foods. And there are indeed specific manufacturers of some food products included in the listings. Where there happens to be more than one manufacturer for a particular food, it is important to locate the listing for the manufacturer of the food product you are researching. You need specific information about specific products, and that specific information includes who manufactures the product. Different manufacturers have different recipes, and every ingredient is important.

Scientists testing glycemic index of foods listed Kellogg's Corn Flakes in the 2002 International tables of Glycemic Index and Glycemic Load Values.[69] Entry number 168 in the 2002 tables is for Kellogg's Corn Flakes. You can see it for yourself at this link right here, or enter the internet address from the footnote at the bottom of the page. The listed glycemic index of Kellogg's Corn Flakes is 92. That means that those flakes create a glycemic response 92%, nearly as powerful as drinking pure glucose. For a 30 gram serving of Kellogg's Corn Flakes, you get a glycemic load of 24. And those corn flakes are not even "frosted." We will continue our timeline with information you can use on your own journey. Now we'll take a look at a conversation between Anne L. Peters, MD and Jennie Brand-Miller:

NUTRITIONAL PRINCIPLES vs. DRUGS AND INSULIN

In a Medscape article, published June 30, 2015, Jennie Brand-Miller, PhD, who holds a chair in human nutrition in the School of Life and Environmental Sciences at the University of Sydney, and Anne L. Peters, MD were interviewed.

Dr. Peters who has a strong background in nutrition, states "I can help my patients just as much by teaching them nutritional principles (including how and what to eat) as I can by teaching them about drugs and insulin.

Lowering the glycemic index through diet is a nice way of lowering A1C without having to take another pill."[70]

---

[69] https://academic.oup.com/ajcn/article/76/1/5/4689459
[70] Anne L. Peters, MD; Jennie Brand-Miller, PhD "Demystifying the Glycemic Index: Implications for Practice." Medscape. June 30, 2015
Accessed at http://www.medscape.com/viewarticle/846945

During the interview, Brand-Miller tells Peters about a study conducted. It was a 12 week <u>randomized controlled trial.</u> One group consumed a low-fat diet while the other group ate a low-glycemic-index version of that same diet.[71]

Brand-Miller states: "The group on the low-glycemic-index diet saw double the fat mass reduction over 12 weeks.

Over 12 weeks we saw that the latter group lost double the fat mass (about 5 kg instead of 2.5 kg).

They also improved their low-density lipoprotein (LDL) levels. The effects were both cardiovascular and weight-based.

They improved their high-density lipoprotein (HDL) levels as well." [72]

Aren't these the numbers we look at when we weigh our risk factors for heart disease?

GLYCEMIC SUMMIT

Positive and negative health effects based on the *quality,* or the *personality* of carbohydrates in the diet interests not only scientific researchers but is also of great interest to the consumer.

In 2013, a group of about twenty International carbohydrate metabolism experts held a scientific summit on a little island off the coast of Italy.

The summit, called the International Scientific Consensus Summit from the International Carbohydrate Quality Consortium (ICQC) considered controversies surrounding the usefulness of the glycemic index (GI), glycemic load (GL) and glycemic response (GR).

Following detailed review of much scientific research, the team noted the importance of the behavior of blood sugar levels after meals (<u>postprandial glycaemia</u>) in overall health.

---

[71] McMillan-Price J, Petocz P, Atkinson F, et al. " Comparison of 4 diets of varying glycemic load on weight loss and cardiovascular risk reduction in overweight and obese young adults." Arch Intern Med. 2006; 166:1466-1475. Accessed at: https://www.ncbi.nlm.nih.gov/pubmed/16864756

[72] Anne L. Peters, MD; Jennie Brand-Miller, PhD "Demystifying the Glycemic Index: Implications for Practice." Medscape. June 30, 2015
Accessed at http://www.medscape.com/viewarticle/846945

Scientists follow the scientific method to validate their work. One requirement of the scientific method is that the same results will be reproduced at another time with another group of people, given the same set of conditions. This team of scientists agreed that, indeed, "The GI is a compelling and reproducible method of classifying carbohydrate foods for the purpose of understanding *postprandial glycaemia.*" [73]

They went on to clarify that, "Overall, the dietary GI seems to be the strongest risk factor for T2DM while GL for heart disease.... Given essentially conclusive evidence that high GI/GL diets contribute to risk of T2DM and CVD [cardio-vascular disease], reduction in GI and GL should be a public health priority. The expert panel confirmed an urgent need to communicate information on GI and GL to the general public and health professionals, through channels such as national dietary guidelines, food composition tables and food labels."[74]

And as we've already discussed, these experts also note that "Moderate to weak *associations* were observed for selected cancers."[75]

---

[73] Augustin L, Kendall C, Jenkins D, et al. "Glycemic index, glycemic load and glycemic response: An International Scientific Consensus Summit from the International Carbohydrate Quality Consortium (ICQC)". Nutr Metab Cardiovasc Dis. 2015 Sep; 25(9):795-815. Doi: 10.1016/j.numecd.2015.05.005. Epub 2015 May 16.
Also Accessed 10-02-16 at https://www.ncbi.nlm.nih.gov/pubmed/26160327
And http://www.nmcd-journal.com/article/S0939-4753(15)00127-1/abstract
[74] Augustin L, Kendall C, Jenkins D, et al. "Glycemic index, glycemic load and glycemic response: An International Scientific Consensus Summit from the International Carbohydrate Quality Consortium (ICQC)." Nutr Metab Cardiovasc Dis. 2015 Sep; 25(9):795-815. Doi: 10.1016/j.numecd.2015.05.005. Epub 2015 May 16.
Abstract Accessed 10-02-16 at: https://www.ncbi.nlm.nih.gov/pubmed/26160327
Full text document accessed 10-04-16 at: http://www.nmcd-journal.com/article/S0939-4753(15)00127-1/fulltext
[75] Ibid.

PART 3: WHY YOU NEED GLYCEMIC LOAD

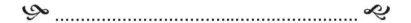

L et's say you're a patient who just left your Dr's office with a diagnosis of pre-diabetes. Although that diagnosis could just as easily be cancer, depression, insulin resistance, low HDL & high LDL levels, or even heart disease, for the sake of this discussion, we will look at receiving a diagnosis of pre-diabetes from a patients' perspective.

You feel scared and confused. You know that some of the foods you are eating are causing distress to your body somehow, but you really don't know how. You don't even know where to begin. You thought you were doing a pretty good job taking care of your health. But you did notice that lately your energy levels haven't been quite what they used to be.

Your doctor mentioned blood sugar levels, and he mentioned carbohydrates. You really don't want to wait for six months to find out if the situation improves itself just by watching your diet. Heck, you're not even sure what to watch for.

So you head over to a discount book store to find some new recipe books and save a bit of money in the process. When you look at the large selection of cookbooks available, you might be thinking, "There are masses of *Glycemic Index, Diabetic, Weight Loss, and Carb Counting* recipe books." Not really sure where to begin, you decide that the "diabetes" category is your best bet since your diagnosis is pre-diabetes. You tentatively pick out half a dozen nice looking books with recipes for managing type 2 diabetes.

Examining your potential selections, you focus on some nice looking diabetic recipe books with really pretty pictures of food. These books were written by the American Diabetes Association. You dread the thought of poking yourself with a needle several times a day to test blood samples. It makes you squeamish to even consider injecting yourself with insulin. Your goal is to reverse that pre-diabetes diagnosis before your next Dr. appointment in six months.

Inside the books you find some seemingly helpful Food Exchange Lists, a few charts and maybe some diagrams on how to build a healthy plate for yourself. It looks like reversing that pre-diabetes diagnosis in six months will be easy and delicious at the same time!

The problem with the Food Exchange schemes is that they are not even just the very tip of the iceberg of the information you really need for blood sugar control. These food lists that have been around since before 1976, and they have been revised at least three times already, while the number of type 2 diabetics have soared.

The Food Exchange lists measure the *amount* of carbohydrate in foods and allow you to interchange among the various items on each list, but do not recognize the effect of the glycemic index of those foods. Has this been effective? It has been effective to a certain degree in helping type 2 diabetics regulate external insulin. But we have watched as our population has embarked on an epidemic of type 2 diabetes, depression, heart disease, and cancer. And so you may start to realize that the term diabetic diet is fraught with much misunderstanding and confusion.

What you really need is the glycemic index scores of foods and their carbohydrate content so that you can calculate the glycemic load. But at this point, you've never even heard of a glycemic index. So we will definitely get into these details later. In the meantime, back to your quest.

Here you are struggling to understand how to deal with your new diagnosis. This is ALL NEW to you. You figure that they have a lot of experience at the American Diabetes Association. After all, they are the American Diabetes Association! So you take your top selection to the register. You make your purchase, take your book home, and stick to the food exchange lists and the diagrams showing you how to build your plate.

Six months later, when you see your Dr., your A1C level is even a bit higher. You have officially tipped into the range of type 2 diabetes. Shocked by the news after all your hard work, you receive a prescription for Metformin, and a recommendation to attend a diabetes support group in your area.

When you get home, you go the American Diabetes Association (ADA) website looking for answers. Right away you see ads for blood glucose test supplies, information on how to use them, and a lot of other information about complications that can happen if you do not take better care of yourself. But you thought you did take better care of yourself by following the ADA diet.

SCIENTIFIC MEASURES TO BODILY RESPONSES

Anyone who is trying to figure out why they have heart disease, cancer, depression, insulin resistance, pre-diabetes or type 2 diabetes really needs information about the carbohydrates that don't spike their blood sugar levels. The only reliable way to assure that is to know *how high* different carbohydrate foods will cause blood sugar levels to go. Luckily we have the International Tables of GI/GL. Scientists who studied the effects of thousands of carbohydrates on human test subjects created these tables just for people to use to manage their blood sugar levels. Everything else really is really just guesswork.

So, the first problem with your books from the American Diabetes Association (ADA) is that the glycemic index is <u>not</u> included for any of the carbohydrate choices listed in those groups of food. To get a closer look at the problem, we'll take a look at a screenshot and some tables to compare information provided by the ADA to the information available in the International Tables of GI/GL.

Here is a screenshot taken from the American Diabetes Association website, showing the information they offer on glycemic index:

Low GI Foods (55 or less)

- 100% stone-ground whole wheat or pumpernickel bread
- Oatmeal (rolled or steel-cut), oat bran, muesli
- Pasta, converted rice, barley, bulgar
- Sweet potato, corn, yam, lima/butter beans, peas, legumes and lentils
- Most fruits, non-starchy vegetables and carrots

Medium GI (56-69)

- Whole wheat, rye and pita bread
- Quick oats
- Brown, wild or basmati rice, couscous

High GI (70 or more)

- White bread or bagel
- Corn flakes, puffed rice, bran flakes, instant oatmeal
- Shortgrain white rice, rice pasta, macaroni and cheese from mix
- Russet potato, pumpkin
- Pretzels, rice cakes, popcorn, saltine crackers
- melons and pineapple

[76, 77]

The first problem with this list is that it doesn't list the actual glycemic index, a most important piece of data for each food. This list just places foods somewhere in the low, medium, or high range of the glycemic index scale. How can we see where, exactly, a specific food is on the glycemic index? From the list above, we certainly can't. As you read on, you will understand why this is so important.

---

[76] http://www.diabetes.org/food-and-fitness/food/what-can-i-eat/understanding-carbohydrates/glycemic-index-and-diabetes.html   Screenshot taken 9-26-16

[77] https://www.diabetes.org/glycemic-index-and-diabetes Information verified as current as of 4-21-20

What makes this simplistic scheme worse for any user is that the "medium" range for glycemic index spans 13 points. This leaves a wide area of great risk for anyone seeking to effectively control their blood sugar levels. Every glycemic index point counts when calculating glycemic load.

Here is an image that provides the actual ranges for low, medium, and high glycemic index; and low, medium, and high glycemic load:

Glycemic Index and Glycemic Load Rankings

Glycemic Index:
Low: 0 – 55
Medium: 56 – 69
High: 70+

Glycemic Load:
Low: 0 – 10
Medium: 11 – 19
High: 20 +

In order to compare the items the American Diabetes Association (ADA) reports have a low glycemic index, we'll compare them with the scientifically tested – on human test subjects – glycemic values reported in the International Tables of Glycemic Index and Glycemic Load. For a food to be low glycemic, we need to see a rank of 55 or less in those international tables. The food also must have a glycemic load of 10 or less. We'll start with the first entry they consider to be low glycemic, 100% stone-ground whole wheat or pumpernickel bread.

BREAD

In order to verify the ADA data that 100% stone-ground whole wheat or pumpernickel bread actually has a low glycemic index as tested on human test subjects, we need to see proof of a glycemic index of 55 or less in order to be truly low glycemic index. And most importantly, we will be looking for a glycemic load (GL) of 10 or less (in the right column) to be truly low glycemic load. In the table below, we can see what the International Tables of Glycemic Index and Glycemic Load report as actual low glycemic index & low glycemic load breads available in the USA. Keep in mind that all of the breads included in the International Tables have been scientifically tested on human test subjects. The serving sizes are measured in grams:

Ref #	Food	GI	Gram Serv	Avail Carb	GL
260	Healthy Choice™ Hearty 7 Grain (Con Agra Inc, USA)	55	30	14	8
261	Healthy Choice™ Hearty 100% Whole Grain (Con Agra Inc., USA)	62	30	14	9
139	Muesli bread, made from packet mix in bread maker (Con Agra Inc., USA)	54	30	12	7
274	Nutty Natural ™ whole grain bread (Natural Ovens, USA)	59	30	12	7
281	Soy & Linseed bread made from packet mix in bread maker (Con Agra Inc., USA)	50	30	10	5
289	100% Whole Grain™ bread (Natural Ovens, USA)	51	30	13	7

[78]

That's it folks. You can view the 2008 tables here,[79] and look under the "Bread" category to see if your brand has been tested and is listed. Breads begin at #101 in the tables and go through #296. There are 195 different breads that have been tested on human subjects. That's a lot of dough.

You can see that "Healthy Choice™" and "Natural Ovens™" each offer two choices that have been human tested and deliver a low glycemic load of 10 or less for a 30g serving. There are also two qualifying breads (produced by Con Agra that you bake from a package. And that 30g serving is about one slice of bread.

So, out of all of those shelves, stocked to the ceiling with so many loaves, there may be essentially four breads to choose from. That is, if in fact they are available in your store at all. And if you include the two package mixes to be made in a bread machine, we come up with six breads.

---

[78] https://www.ncbi.nlm.nih.gov/pmc/articles/PMC2584181/
[79] http://care.diabetesjournals.org/content/diacare/suppl/2008/09/18/dc08-1239.DC1/TableA1_1.pdf

If you want to make a sandwich, a Romaine lettuce leaf or two make a good top if your goal is to maintain a low glycemic index/load and still eat bread. (And better yet, to be certain – or to get faster results, you could skip the bread and just use Collard greens, Romaine lettuce, Swiss chard, or another leafy green to replace the bread entirely.)

Now, if you think you have located a 100% whole wheat bread at your grocer, be sure to read the ingredient label to be sure that you see 100% whole wheat or pumpernickel listed as the very first ingredient.

Bread made from 100% whole grains will be heavy rather than the light and fluffy stuff commonly called bread and stacked to the ceiling in the grocery aisles. You will also be able to see those whole grains right there in the loaf. This bread will be chewy rather than fluffy. And it will keep you feeling full longer. If not available at your grocer, a health food store might carry a true 100% stone ground whole wheat bread.

A review of the pumpernickel breads in the www.glycemicindex.com database and the International Tables of GI/GL 2008 show a total of only four pumpernickel breads that have a low GI and a low GL. Those four pumpernickel breads are made in Canada, not in the US. Won't it be wonderful when the American Diabetes Association provides accurate information for foods available to those that live in the country they represent?

So unless you are selecting a pumpernickel loaf with seeds you can actually see, and with 100% whole grain listed as the first ingredient, there is currently NO WAY you can be sure it is low GI/GL. Many "pumpernickel" breads are pumped up into fluffy loaves with the addition of highly refined grains (like wheat or white flour) by manufacturers and clearly jump right out of the low glycemic range.

PASTA

The ADA also puts pasta in their low glycemic category. To be low glycemic, the food needs a GI score of 55 or less. Pasta and Noodles begin at 1325 and end at 1388 in the 2008 tables, for a total of 60 entries. There are only two scientifically tested pastas that are manufactured in the USA available in the results. Both of them meet the requirement of being 55 or under on the GI scale, but both of them are over the low glycemic load limit of 10 for a 180 g serving. Neither one of the two qualifying pastas are found at the grocery store.

If you review the 2008 tables for Pasta, you will notice that except for entry #1360, they all have a 180g serving size, or about 6 1/3 oz. You may notice that several really do have a low glycemic index compared to glucose (the first column on the left marked GI at the top). But not a single one of them has a low glycemic load (the last column on the right).

Can you find a number that is 10 or less in the right-hand column for ANY pasta entry scientifically tested on human subjects -- anywhere in the international tables?

I know it is hard to read those tables. So here is a simple table of the tested USA pastas for you that have a low glycemic index, but at that 180 g typical serving size, neither one of them has a low glycemic load:

Ref #	FOOD	GI	SERV SIZE	Avail Carb	GL
1351	Proti pasta, protein enriched, boiled in water (Vital Nature, Inc, San Antonio, USA)	28	180	49	14
1362	Spaghetti, soy (Revival Soy®, Physicians Pharmaceuticals, Inc USA)	47	180	37	17

[80]

That's it folks. Looking at the 180g serving size, you would have to cut that in half in order to have a low glycemic load. That would give you 90g or about 3 ounces of pasta.

In an effort to save us time and space, here is a basic summary of my general findings on pasta and rice:

---

[80] https://www.ncbi.nlm.nih.gov/pmc/articles/PMC2584181/

Noodling out the Best Pasta?

Pasta	Glycemic Index	Grams Serving	Carbs	Glycemic Load
Spaghetti	46	180	47	22
Lasagna	55	180	47	26
Corn	63	180	46	31
Buckwheat	59	180	42	35
Rice	92	180	49	35
Buttery Rice	79	150	49	40

[81]

So about the only way to eat pasta or rice is to cut the typical serving size in half or even thirds. In the case of Buttery Rice, you might consider only a quarter. It is not even close to a food that can be considered "low glycemic." The first entry is spaghetti, with a glycemic load of 22. So much for the glycemic index of 46, that serving is going to spike your blood sugar. If you cut that serving of spaghetti in half, your glycemic load still comes in at 11, and that is no longer a low glycemic load, either. This is one example of why using only the glycemic index of a food can be ineffective to control blood sugar.

POTATOES

SWEET POTATOES AND YAMS

Next, we'll look at a table created to present an overview of the information listed in the International Tables of GI/GL Values 2008 for Sweet Potatoes Sweet potatoes are another entry on the ADA list of "Low Glycemic Index" foods. Notice that some sweet potatoes do indeed have a low glycemic index, but none of them have a low glycemic load:

SWEET POTATOES
GLYCEMIC INDEX, CARBOHYDRATE & GLYCEMIC LOAD

Ref #	Country of Origin	GI	Gram Serv	Carbs	GL
1684	Australia	44	150	25	11
1685	Jamaica	46	150	32	15
1686	Australia	61	150	18	11
1687	New Zealand	77	150	25	19
1688	Jamaica	94	150	45	42
1689	Jamaica	76	150	45	34
1690	Jamaica	82	150	45	37
1691	China	77	150	21	16
1692	Australia	75	150	29	21

[82]

I hope you are beginning to see the truth about the sweet potato and yam that are next on the list of low glycemic index foods at the American Diabetes Association website. Hopefully you are beginning to realize how the "low," medium," and "high" designations can really mess up your efforts at blood sugar control.

Next we'll look at a representative sampling of Yams. The serving sizes are measured in grams:

---

[82] https://www.ncbi.nlm.nih.gov/pmc/articles/PMC2584181/

YAMS
GLYCEMIC INDEX, CARBOHYDRATE & GLYCEMIC LOAD

Ref #	Country of Origin	GI	Serv	Carbs	GL
1697	New Zealand	35	150	36	13
1698	China	54	150	36	19
1700	Nigeria	76	150	38	28
1704	Jamaica	77	150	38	29
1706	Jamaica	73	150	39	28
1707	Jamaica	68	150	34	23
1710	Jamaica	82	150	39	32

[83]

If you are in New Zealand, Australia, Jamaica, or China, you might actually find a sweet potato or a yam with a low *glycemic index* ranking. But at a 150g (or about 5 ¼ oz.) serving, you are not going to find a sweet potato or yam with a low *glycemic load* anywhere in the world!

Sweet potato and yam contain more vitamins and minerals than white potatoes. But a portion *much* smaller than 5 ½ oz. – less than half of the listed amount *might* be considered feasible in a low glycemic load meal. And as you can see, much depends on where that yam grew up! Preparation methods may also make a difference, and we will look at some possible options when we look at The Resistant Starch Solution.

It is unfortunate that our country did not provide sweet potato or yam for glycemic index testing. But we can see how these foods affect human test subjects in other countries, and use that as a clue. And in the typical serving sizes, no one will escape a blood sugar

---

[83] https://www.ncbi.nlm.nih.gov/pmc/articles/PMC2584181/

spike. So if we are trying to control blood sugar levels, we might like to have only a very small portion.

WHITE POTATOES

The ADA website shows Russet potatoes to have a high GI (which is 70 or above). But there are a few things about potatoes that you'll want to know. The 2008 tables have 56 results for white potatoes, numbering from 1627 through 1683. Here is a basic Spud List:

Keeping an Eye on the Spud

Potato	Glycemic Index	Grams Serving	Carbs	Glycemic Load
Russet	111	150	30	33
Red	89	150	21	19
Instant Mashed (mean 6)	87	150	20	17
Ore-Ida® Fries	64	150	32	21

[84]

If you review the GI and GL numbers for all of the potatoes, you will find one acceptable potato, in a typical serving size, in the entire international collection. The entry is # 1654. This particular potato was boiled in salted water, refrigerated for 24 hours, and reheated. It has a GI of only 23, a 150g serving, 34g of carbs, just like the others, and a GL of only 8. Now, that is acceptable.

But you're not receiving it at a fast food drive thru window, or at a restaurant. As you can see, much depends on how the potato is prepared. And after looking at entry # 1654, you can see that there is a way to prepare the potato that lowers glycemic impact, and we will return to that subject in a moment. But first, while we are on the subject of potatoes, we'll

---

[84] https://www.ncbi.nlm.nih.gov/pmc/articles/PMC2584181/

look at an eye-opening study about the highly promoted, readily available French fry and what researchers have learned about its extensive worldwide consumption.

The March 2016 issue of Diabetes Care published a study which reviewed dietary information on over 199,000 U.S. male and female health professionals without cancer, cardiovascular disease, or diabetes at the beginning of the research period. They report that "greater concurrent and increased potato consumption was associated with a higher risk for T2D…. Moreover, increased consumption of French fries was positively associated with subsequent T2D risk…. The positive associations observed in this analysis further corroborate the hypothesis that increased potato intake may lead to an increased risk for T2D." [85] Notice how often we consider "associations" when we look at scientific research.

These researchers looked at how many potatoes the study participants had eaten over a four year time period. They looked at who reported getting a diagnosis of diabetes during that time. It turned out that the more potatoes these subjects ate, especially French fries, the greater chance they had of getting type 2 diabetes. This was true in spite of BMI (body mass index) and any other risk factors. This is the first of its kind look into the potato, classified as a healthful vegetable under the USDA "My Plate" National Guidelines of Healthy Eating.

Let's hope this review of nearly *two hundred thousand people* casts serious doubt about the potato remaining in a healthful vegetable category here in the U.S.A. In the U.K. the potato is placed in the cereal group, which more clearly reflects its impact on blood sugar levels.

THE RESISTANT STARCH SOLUTION

Potatoes fill us up, stretch our food budget, and are often considered a "comfort food."

The problem is that potatoes are mainly starch, and normal starch is so easy to digest. Those cookies, muffins, cakes, pastas, breads, donuts, pastries are also mainly starch, and easy to digest. During digestion, starches are quickly converted to glucose and absorbed by our cells, sending blood sugar levels high (hyperglycemia).

When blood sugar levels get high, our pancreas produces insulin to bring them down again. The higher our blood sugar levels get, the more insulin our body produces to send the extra glucose into our cells. If our tissues do not need the glucose for energy, that glucose is stored as fat. Sending glucose to our tissues can lower blood sugar levels

---

[85] Muraki I, Rimm E, Willett W. "Potato Consumption and Risk of Type 2 Diabetes: Results From Three Prospective Cohort Studies." Diabetes Care 2016 Mar; 39(3): 376-384. http://dx.doi.org/10.2337/dc15-0547 Accessed 10-19-16

dramatically, and even result in <u>hypoglycemia</u>. "Repetition of this hyper- and hypoglycemic cycle appears to result in insulin resistance and type 2 diabetes, thereby contributing to obesity."[86]

But there is another way to prepare potatoes that does not have such a profound negative effect. Converting the simple starch of the potato into a "resistant" starch holds much hope for the potato loving among us.

"According to numerous previous studies it could be concluded that resistant starch can reduce fat accumulation, enhance insulin sensitivity, regulate blood glucose level and lipid metabolism. Recent investigations have focused on the possible associations between resistant starch and incretins as well as gut microbiota. Resistant starch seems to be a promising dietary fiber for the prevention or treatment of obesity and its related diseases." [87]

"In human subjects, insulin sensitivity is *increased* with the feeding of resistant starch."[88] Remember we looked at the scientific test results of one potato that was boiled in salted water, refrigerated overnight, and then reheated? For the same 150g serving as any other potato entry, that one particular potato had a glycemic index of only 23 and a glycemic load of 8. But do keep in mind that it still contains 34 g of carbohydrate.

Let's say you are dosing external insulin based on carb counts alone. You are checking your blood sugar levels an hour after meals to see if you need to inject more insulin. At that one hour check, you will want to note of the impact of resistant starch on your blood sugar level. You want to compare it to the impact you noted for non-resistant starch (freshly prepared potatoes) and perhaps make adjustments to the amount of insulin you require.

Now we'll take a look at a table of the different types of resistant starch:

[86] Birt D, Boylston T, Hendrich S, et al. "Resistant Starch: Promise for Improving Human Health." Adv Nutr November 2013 Adv Nutr vol. 4: 587-601, 2013. doi: 10.3945/?an.113.004325 Accessed on 10-20-16 at: http://advances.nutrition.org/content/4/6/587.full

[87] Zhang L, Li HT, Shen L, et al. "Effect of Dietary Resistant Starch on Prevention and Treatment of Obesity-related Diseases and Its Possible Mechanisms." Biomed Environ Sci. 2015 Apr; 28(4):291-7. Doi: 10.3967/bes2015.040. Accessed 11-01-16 at https://www.ncbi.nlm.nih.gov/pubmed/25966755.
[88] Keenan M, Zhou J, Hegsted M, et al. "Role of resistant starch in improving gut health, adiposity, and insulin resistance." Adv Nutr. 2015 Mar 13;6(2):198-205. Doi: 10.3945/an.114.007419. Accessed 10-21-16 at: https://www.ncbi.nlm.nih.gov/pubmed/25770258

TABLE 1
Types of resistant starches[1]

Designation	Description	Example	Referenc
RSI	Physically inaccessible starch	Coarsely ground or whole-kernel grains	(1)
RSII	Granular starch with the B- or C-polymorph	High-amylose maize starch, raw potato, raw banana starch	(1)
RSIII	Retrograded starch	Cooked and cooled starchy foods	(24)
RSIV	Chemically modified starches	Cross-linked starch and octenyl succinate starch	(25)
RSV	Amylose-lipid complex	Stearic acid-complexed high-amylose starch	(31)

1   RSI, type I resistant starch; (RS); RSII, type II resistant starch; RSIII, type III resistant starch; RS
     type IV resistant starch; RSV; type V resistant starch.

89

In the above image, you can see that a physically inaccessible starch, such as whole or coarsely ground grains is classified as Resistant Starch I. That's because these grain kernels are enclosed in bran, the high fiber component of the grain. The bran makes the large endosperm portion of the grain less available to the forces of digestion.

In Resistant Starch II, the example given is raw potato or raw banana. These are resistant to digestion because they are not cooked. And this is also true for pasta, and the degree to which it is cooked. For example, al dente pasta, by virtue of its shortened boiling time, has a lower glycemic index than tender pasta that has boiled for 20 minutes. Shortened cooking time also lowers the glycemic load of the pasta (al dente), because it has a lower glycemic index.

Resistant starch III is retrograded starch. It has been cooked and cooled before serving. For instance, preparing a potato salad and refrigerating it overnight before serving lowers the glycemic index of the pasta. A working example of creating this type of starch is found in potato entry Ref #1652. This spud has a GI of 88, GL of 18. The same freshly boiled and served spud has a GI of 118, GL of 24 (entry Ref #1646.) When we compare the two,

---

we can see that when the pasta was cooked and refrigerated 24 hrs. before consuming, the GI dropped down to 88 from 118. That's 30 points less in terms of glycemic index. And the glycemic load fell from 24 to 18. While it's not a low glycemic load, it's still 6 points lower than it was before the 24 hour refrigeration. This treatment also applies to the prepared, refrigerated, mashed potatoes and pasta salads sold in some deli departments. But do keep in mind serving sizes.

A technique to reduce glycemic index even further is to boil the potato, cool and refrigerate overnight, then reheat just before serving, as represented in entry Ref #1654. This spud has a GI of 23, GL of only 6. The same spud (entry Ref #1649) when boiled and served fresh has a GI of 76, GL of 26. But when refrigerated for 24 hours and reheated just before serving, we drop 53 points on the GI and 20 points on the GL. (Be sure to apply safe food handling measures, such as cooling quickly and refrigerating as soon as possible.)

POPCORN

This time I'd like to show you another disagreement between the scientific test results in the International Tables of GI/GL Values 2008, and the ADA Glycemic Index Food List.

The ADA classifies popcorn as a high glycemic food. Popcorn is a whole grain. It's popped, but all of its nutrition is intact. Nothing has been removed by refining or processing. Let's take a look at what the 2008 tables have to say about popcorn:

POPCORN
GLYCEMIC INDEX, CARBOHYDRATE & GLYCEMIC LOAD

Ref #	Country of Origin	GI	Serv.	Carbs	GL
1451	Canada	72	20 g.	12	9
1453	Canada	58	20 g.	12	7
1453	China	55	20 g.	10	6
1454	Australia	55	20 g.	11	6
1455	Australia	62	20 g.	10	6
1456	Australia	67	20 g.	11	10
1457	Australia	89	20 g.	11	7

[90]

While popcorn may have a high glycemic index, (as high as 70 and above) in a few cases, you will notice that it has a low glycemic load (of 10 or less) in *every* case. This is another example of why glycemic index does not tell the whole story about a foods effect on blood sugar levels. You may also notice that popcorn contains only 10 – 12 grams of carbohydrate in about a 2 cup serving of popped kernels.

Popcorn is a lovely snack, because it retains its bran, germ and is loaded with fiber. You can go ahead and eat about 20 g. of popcorn and still have a low glycemic load at the end of your snack. [91] [92]

Watermelon is a another example of a high glycemic index fruit (GI of about 75) but a low glycemic load of only about 4 for a 120g. (about ½ cup) serving. So go ahead and enjoy a

---

[90] https://www.ncbi.nlm.nih.gov/pmc/articles/PMC2584181/
[91] http://www.health.harvard.edu/diseases-and-conditions/glycemic_index_and_glycemic_load_for_100_foods
[92] and http://www.glycemicindex.com/foodSearch.php

nice cold slice on a hot summer day! [93] [94]

FOOD EXCHANGE PERILS

This book would not be complete without a comparison of some *Food Exchanges* from the American Diabetes Association (ADA) and the actual tests of glycemic index on human subjects for those foods. In the top half of the next image you can see an ADA "fruit exchange." In the first example, a banana is compared to a pear, because they are treated equally in the ADA "fruit list." The next is what is deemed a "starch exchange." For the starch exchange we compare a slice of white bread to a half cup of lentil soup. The following image includes the actual scientifically tested glycemic index rankings of these foods for you:

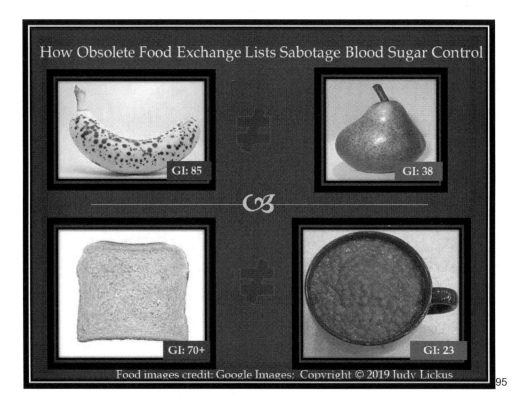

[95]

Remember The Glycemic Index and Glycemic Load Range from Low to High. Here is an image of glycemic index rankings:

---

[93] http://www.health.harvard.edu/diseases-and-conditions/glycemic_index_and_glycemic_load_for_100_foods
[94] and http://www.glycemicindex.com/foodSearch.php
[95] https://www.ncbi.nlm.nih.gov/pmc/articles/PMC2584181/

```
Glycemic Index:
Low: 0 – 55
Medium: 56 – 69
High: 70+
```

Using the above glycemic index table to recognize high, medium, and low glycemic foods, you take another look at how the banana and the pear rank on their glycemic index (GI) scores included in the above graphic. See how far apart these two fruits are in their glycemic index (GI)? The difference between the glycemic indexes of these two fruits is 47 points.

Next, consider the slice of white bread compared to the bowl of lentil soup in the lower portion of the ADA graphic we looked at earlier. Using the above table as your new lens again, you find that the bread and the lentil soup are not at all similar in glycemic index. They are not even close. There is a difference of 47 points minimum, depending on the type of bread. Can you see why they are not equal in terms of how high they raise blood sugar levels when people eat them?

Back to you, your diagnosis, and the book you trusted to help you reverse that diagnosis. I hope you begin to realize what is wrong with that book, and why those "Food Exchange" lists have earned you the diagnosis of type 2 diabetes.

You may as well celebrate by having a slice of cake, because a slice of cake may very well have a lower GI/GL than a slice of white bread, ounce for ounce. Really. We'll begin the next chapter with a closer look at how a slice of bread and a slice of cake compare in their glycemic load scores.

FOOD SCIENCE IN THE KITCHEN

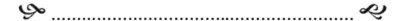

T he image below shows the number of carbs in a 30 g. (about one ounce) serving of bread and a 30 g. (about one ounce) serving of cake. It also shows the glycemic index of each, and how we calculate the glycemic load for the bread and the cake:

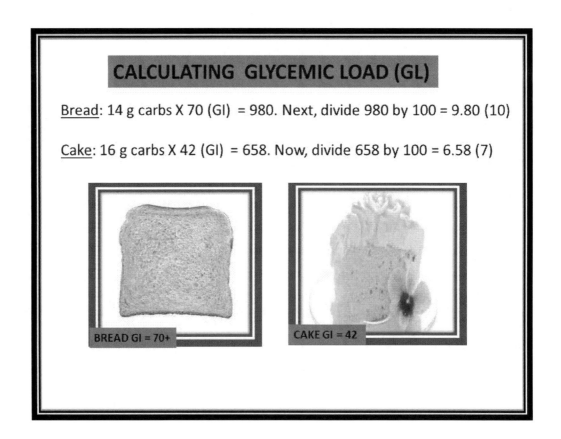

CALCULATING GLYCEMIC LOAD (GL)

Bread: 14 g carbs X 70 (GI) = 980. Next, divide 980 by 100 = 9.80 (10)

Cake: 16 g carbs X 42 (GI) = 658. Now, divide 658 by 100 = 6.58 (7)

BREAD GI = 70+

CAKE GI = 42

While a serving of the cake may have two more carbs than the slice of bread, the cake has a low glycemic index. The bread, on the other hand, has a high glycemic index. When you multiply the number of carbs by the GI score to calculate the glycemic load, you get a much higher number for the bread (980) than you do for the cake (658). When you divide each of these numbers by 100, you get 9.8 (rounded up to 10) for the bread, and 6.6 (rounded up to 7) for the cake.

Here's a real-life example: Let's say you are administering additional insulin based on carb counts. In that case, you might increase your dose for the cake because of the higher carb count. But because the cake would not raise your blood sugar as much as the bread, it becomes possible to create the medical error of hypoglycemia. That can happen because your blood sugar does not, in fact, rise as high when eating the cake as it does when eating the bread.

WORKING WITH GLYCEMIC VALUES

One of the first things we want to look at are assigned values. For some foods, the carbohydrate content was so low that the volunteer test subjects were unable to eat a portion containing 50 g. of carbohydrate. Another issue is that not all food products received testing. For these foods, the researchers "assigned" a GI value. The assigned values are for the basic food, without being a part of a recipe. These assigned values may be easy to remember and help in your selection process. But use caution because, for example, yogurt is a dairy product, but many manufactured yogurt products often have much added sugar. Here is an image showing the assigned GI values of three types of basic foods, dairy, vegetable, and flour:

Assigned GI Values for Unlisted Foods

Food	Assigned GI Value
Dairy Product	30
Vegetable	40
Flour products	70

[96]

---

[96] Atkinson F, Foster-Powell K, Brand-Miller J. "International tables of Glycemic Index and Glycemic Load Values: 2008." *Diabetes Care*. December; 31(12): 2281-2283. Doi: 10.2337/dc08-1239. Retrieved from: http://www.ncbi.nlm.nih.gov/pmc/articles/PMC2584181/

Assigned GI values can be helpful especially when you don't have access to the actual glycemic values of specific foods.

Other foods were found to have no glycemic index at all. In order to test glycemic index, 50 g. carbohydrate servings are necessary. Some foods just don't contain enough carbohydrate, and some foods are made up of mainly the fiber component of carbohydrate (like avocadoes), while others contain no or very little carbohydrate. These foods include eggs, fish, meat, nuts, poultry, seeds, tofu, some fruits (especially berries), and salad vegetables. These foods do not affect your blood sugar levels and so they have no glycemic index.

When we look at the Assigned GI value of 70 for flour products, we realize that most breads, cookies, doughnuts, pancakes, waffles, bagels, and buns are made from flour products. And that is only the GI of the flour. After that you factor in the carbohydrate content. When you multiply the amount of carbohydrate by the glycemic index of that carbohydrate, if you get a number greater than 1,000, it no longer has a low glycemic load. Maybe you see why there really aren't any low glycemic load foods made with any flour products. The only way to safely eat any untested flour products is to limit their consumption to a single bite or two in order to avoid a significant spike in blood sugar.

Our smartest work, then is to learn to calculate the glycemic load (GL) so we can manage all the temptations in our lives. Here is another way to look at the process:

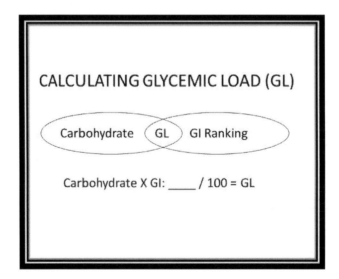

CALCULATING GLYCEMIC LOAD (GL)

Carbohydrate GL GI Ranking

Carbohydrate X GI: _____ / 100 = GL

DELICIOUS BEVERAGES

By now we are mainly aware that canned sodas are an unhealthy choice. Thank goodness those aren't our only options! And what if you are not at home to mix up your own personal favorite? For example, if you are traveling on an airplane, it is common for the flight attendant to offer you a beverage. Popular selections are cranberry juice cocktail, orange juice, tomato juice, or a carbonated beverage such as Coca Cola®, Sprite®, Fanta®, water, tea, or coffee.

Water, tea, and coffee do not have a glycemic index. So they don't raise blood sugar levels.

The next group of beverages images we will look at offer practice in calculating glycemic load.

The images include pictures of glasses filled with different beverages (provided by Google Images). While you can see examples of these popular beverages, here's what else you can see for each beverage in the images below:

1. The amount of carbohydrate (Carbs),
2. The glycemic index (GI)
3. The calculation for glycemic load (GL) of a typical serving size, 250 ml. or about 8 ½ oz.:

Drinking it Up: Beverages 250 ml. Servings

Ocean Spray®
Cranberry Juice
Cocktail

Carbs: 35
GI: 68

Here's the
math:
35 X 68 = 2380
2380 / 100 =
23.80GL

100% Orange
Juice

Carbs: 24
GI: 50

Here's the math:
24 X 50 = 1200
1200 / 100 =
12.00GL

Google Images

Beverages, 250 ml. Cont'd.

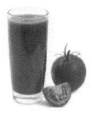

Tomato Juice

Carbs: 8
GI: 33

Here's the math:
8 X 33 = 264
264 / 100 = 2.64GL

Google Image

Carbonated Beverages 250 ml. serving

Coca Cola®

Carbs: 26
GI: 63

Here's the math:
26 X 63 = 1638
1638/100 = 16.38 GL

Fanta®

Carbs: 34
GI: 62

Here's the math:
34 X 62 = 2108
2108/100 = 21.08 GL

Plain Seltzer Water

Carbs: 0
GI: 0

No math to do:
Add a tsp. of any extract for the
flavor you prefer and a few drops of
Liquid Stevia to sweeten.
Suggestions: vanilla, orange,
almond, etc.

Plain Water

Carbs:0
GI: 0

Drink at least
8 glasses each day

Google Image

Always drink plenty of water every day. Start with two glasses when you wake up in the morning. Drink another glass or two a half an hour before each meal. Have another glass about forty minutes after each meal. The goal, for most

GLYCEMIC LOAD FOOD GUIDE & PERSONAL WORKBOOK

adults is to drink nearly a gallon of water, just plain refreshing water, each and every day.

You know you need to drink more water if you ever feel thirsty, or have "dry lips." If you ever feel "thirsty," it means you are already dehydrated. Drink more water. Water is the only thing that will really quench your thirst.

Eliminate table sugar from your home. Start by leaving it out of your coffee or tea. Table sugar is a nasty combination of dextrose (pure glucose) and fructose. Stevia is an easy-to-use sweet substitute that has a negligible effect on blood glucose levels.

It may take 2 or 3 weeks to get over missing the act of stirring in a spoonful of sugar, but once you have kicked that habit you might just wonder what on earth you were ever thinking to add such a thing to compromise the full flavor of your drink!

You might enjoy carbonated beverages. The next time you visit your grocery store, take a look at the extracts in the baking aisle.

Here is a list of extract choices on a neighborhood grocery shelf: Almond, anise, banana, butter, cherry, cinnamon, coconut, hazelnut, orange, peppermint, raspberry, root beer, rum, strawberry, and vanilla. Your store might have even more.

You can replace sugary sodas with plain seltzer water. Add any baking extract of your choice for flavor you enjoy. Sweeteners such as erythritol, stevia, or xylitol can help you create the soft drink of your dreams. This soft drink has virtually no glycemic index and no effect on your blood sugar levels.

Get creative with your ideas and consider ways to lower your glycemic load over the course of each day. Maybe you have the habit of picking up an icy soda at a drive thru restaurant a couple days a week. Perhaps you can ask for plain seltzer water, or how about this idea: Order a glass full of ice. Add your own soda (plain seltzer water), add your own flavoring (one of the baking flavor extracts), and add your own sweetener (stevia works great). Of course you will want to have your ingredients in your vehicle. That means there are a few things less you need to bring into your home after you shop. Keep an extra set of your favorite ingredients for your vehicle. This is how you set yourself up for success. You do what is best for yourself. You will feel much better. And others will respect you more because of it.

But, back to you and your newly found book. No wonder it is so confusing. Not only for you, but for many others who think they will find the answers they need in a book like this. Unfortunately, there are literally tons of books like that. The *Glycemic Index and the Glycemic Load* are missing from most of these books. It really is unfortunate because this is information that has been around for a long time. Using this information could save a lot of people a lot of anguish, but they have to learn about it by themselves. They have to do their own research to even find out that there is this natural way to control blood sugar.

Regarding your search for a good resource, you might even find some books that list the glycemic index of many foods. If you are working with a book that provides only glycemic index, you can find the carbohydrate information you need in the USDA National Nutrient Database file, Food Data Central[97] or on the Nutrition Facts label of a manufactured product. You need to know how many carbs a food contains to calculate the glycemic load. Glycemic load shows you how much of a food to eat and still maintain a low glycemic load to avoid blood sugar spikes and crashes.

To figure the glycemic load, you need the glycemic index and the carb count for your serving size. Then you do your arithmetic. Again, it goes like this:

GI X CARBS: _____ / 100 = GL

Multiply the GI times (X) the number of carbohydrates. Divide that number by 100. That is the glycemic load. When the glycemic load is 10 or less the meal has a low glycemic load, and does not spike blood sugar.

Many people have found calculating glycemic load to be confusing. That's why you have been presented with several examples of calculating glycemic load. Maybe one example makes it easier to understand than another, so that is why they are included.

You really need a reliable system, something you can depend on. You have likely read about some of the complications that can come your way because of uncontrolled blood sugar levels.

And, as you can see, it's not only about type 2 diabetes at all. Sure, the glycemic index came about to help people with diabetes manage their carbohydrate intake. But we have learned, and continue to learn just how much we are affected by our glycemic response. It's just as much about cancer, depression, heart disease, and so many other states of ill-health, as it is about

---

[97] https://fdc.nal.usda.gov/

T2D. You know you don't want to go that way. You know you can do better than that. The simple way to really take control of your health and your future is to do your own arithmetic.

Once you do your own arithmetic, you will know the correct foods to select and the serving sizes to give yourself. You will know the amounts of different foods and beverages to eat that will keep your blood sugar stable. These are the foods you will want to place in your shopping cart to design your meals and build your recipes with. Soon, with practice, you will no longer need to do the arithmetic.

CHARTS FOR CONVERTING METRIC TO US MEASURES

Everything is measured in Metrics for the international tables, but many Americans use Conventional U.S. Measures. Scientists use metrics to measure and report serving sizes when they test foods and beverages for glycemic values. Think about it for a minute. An ounce is equal to twenty eight grams. Think about it another way. It takes twenty eight grams to equal one ounce. That means the mighty gram breaks down an ounce into twenty eight equal parts. When you break an ounce down into twenty eight parts, you can measure a smaller amount and have a plain number without any decimals to "round off" when you do your arithmetic.

In Many Kitchens USA, a measuring cup is frequently used for all ingredients. If you are going to do the job right, and convert metric to US weight measures, you'll need a scale.

But just in case you are not a metric fan, you can still use a simple conversion table until you understand the quantities of different foods you can eat and still maintain a low glycemic load.

The following table shows how different gram measures convert into ounces. The first and third columns list various weights in grams. The second and fourth columns convert the metric weights into ounces.

Maybe now you can picture the number of grams (g.) it takes to weigh in at an ounce (oz.).

METRIC TO U.S. **WEIGHT** CONVERSIONS

GRAMS	OUNCES (rounded)	GRAMS	OUNCES (rounded)
5 g	.18 oz.	80 g	2.82 oz.
10 g	.35 oz.	100 g	3.53 oz.
20 g	.71 oz.	113 g	3.99 oz.
25 g	.88 oz.	120 g	4.23 oz.
28 g	1 oz.	150 g	5.29 oz.
30 g	1.05 oz.	180 g	6.35 oz.
40 g	1.41 oz.	226 g	7.97 oz.
50 g	1.76 oz.	237 g	8.36 oz.
60 g	2.12 oz.	240 g	8.47 oz.
70 g	2.43 oz.	250 g	8.82 oz.

The next table shows how many milliliters (mL) it takes to fill a cup, a fluid ounce (fl. oz.), a tablespoon (Tbsp.), and a teaspoon (Tsp.).

Scientists measure liquids by their volume. Again, as with gram measures, milliliters are much more precise than fluid ounces. It takes 5 mL to measure one liquid teaspoon.

Many measuring cups are marked with both US measures and Metric measures. Purchasing one of these could be a very good investment.

METRIC TO U.S. <u>VOLUME</u> CONVERSIONS

<u>Milliliter</u>	<u>Cup</u>	<u>Fluid Oz</u>	<u>Tbsp.</u>	<u>Tsp.</u>
15 mL	1/16 C	.50 fl. oz.	1Tbsp.	3 Tsp.
30 mL	1/8 C	1 fl. oz.	2 Tbsp.	6 Tsp.
59 mL	1/4 C	2 fl. oz.	4 Tbsp.	12 Tsp.
79 mL	1/3 C	2.75 fl. oz.	5.3 Tbsp.	16 Tsp.
118 mL	1/2 C	4 fl. oz.	8 Tbsp.	24 Tsp.
158 mL	2/3 C	5.50 fl. oz.	10.6 Tbsp.	32 Tsp.
177 mL	3/4 C	6 fl. oz.	12 Tbsp.	36 Tsp.
237 mL	1 C	8 fl. oz.	16 Tbsp.	48 Tsp.
250 mL	1.06 C	8.45 fl. oz.	16.91 Tbsp.	50.72 Tsp.

WEANING YOURSELF OFF OF SUGAR

It really can be hard to escape sugar. Some sugars are fine in moderation, like those that are naturally occurring in most fruits and vegetables. These sugars are often wrapped in fiber, healthy fats and other important nutrients. This means they have a lower glycemic impact.

For example, an avocado is a fruit that is loaded with fiber and monounsaturated fats (the good kind). A one cup serving of this single seeded wonder berry contains 12 g of carbohydrate. But that carbohydrate is made up of 10 g of fiber and only 1g of naturally occurring sugar. When we subtract the 10 g of fiber, we have only 1 g of available carbohydrate. Avocado has "0" glycemic index.

The sugars that are so not fine are those that are "refined" and processed. Other sugars that are not so fine are "added sugars." You have to read the fine print of the "ingredients" list on any food or food-like product to locate these. Actually, you must read the ingredient label on every potential manufactured food-like product that comes in a package with a label!

HOW SWEET IT IS

Table sugar is really a manufactured food product (sucrose) that consists of one half glucose and one half fructose.

Based on the glycemic index alone, you might also think that table sugar, with a GI of about 60 is better than glucose, which has a GI of 100. But what about the fifty percent of fructose used to create that table sugar?

Fructose has a low glycemic index, so when it is combined with glucose to make table sugar (sucrose), the final product, sucrose, has a lower glycemic index than glucose. That sounds great, right? So what is the problem?

GLYCEMIC LOAD FOOD GUIDE & PERSONAL WORKBOOK

WHAT'S WRONG WITH FRUCTOSE?

Vasanti S Malik, ScD, a research scientist, and Frank B Hu, MD, PhD, professor of nutrition and epidemiology, both at the Harvard TH Chan School of Public Health, Boston, Massachusetts conducted an extensive literature review focusing on research conducted on the consumption of sugar-sweetened beverages. Their review was published online in the Journal of the American College of Cardiology in September 28, 2015. This research review was supported by grants from the National Institutes of Health, among others.

Dr.s Malik and Hu see "fructose as having a unique role in the pathogenesis of cardiometabolic diseases." They continue, "However, because we rarely consume fructose in isolation, *the major source of fructose in the diet comes from fructose-containing sugars, sucrose and high fructose corn syrup, in sugar-sweetened beverages and foods.* Intake of sugar-sweetened beverages has been consistently linked to increased risk of obesity, type 2 diabetes, and cardiovascular disease in various populations."[98]

In this article, the authors warn of "incomplete compensation for liquid calories, adverse glycemic effects, and increased hepatic metabolism of fructose leading to de novo lipogenesis [converts excess carbohydrates to fats for storage], production of uric acid, and accumulation of visceral and ectopic fat...and the risk of obesity, diabetes, and cardiovascular disease".[99]

"Indeed, the review reveals that consuming one or two servings a day of sugar-sweetened drinks raises the risk for:

- type 2 diabetes by as much as 26%,
- coronary heart disease by 35%,
- and stroke by 16%.

Weight gain, gout, and kidney disease have been linked to their consumption as well.

While juices may be perceived as healthy because they contain some vitamins and other nutrients, they also contain similar amounts of sugar — albeit natural rather than added — and intake of juice has been associated with weight gain

[98] Malik VS, Hu FB. "Fructose and Cardiometabolic Health what the Evidence from Sugar-Sweetened Beverages Tells Us." *Journal of American Cardiology.* 2015; 66(14):1615-1624. Accessed 9-10-16 at: http://content.onlinejacc.org/article.aspx?articleID=2445331

[99] Malik VS, Hu FB. "Fructose and Cardiometabolic Health what the Evidence from Sugar-Sweetened Beverages Tells Us." *Journal of American Cardiology.* 2015; 66(14):1615-1624. DOI:10.1016/j.jacc.2015.08.025. Accessed 9-10-16 at: http://www.sciencedirect.com/science/article/pii/S0735109715049074

---

and diabetes in some studies. Thus, Dr. Malik says, a maximum of 4 to 6 oz. a day has been recommended."[100]

UPDATED DIETARY GUIDELINES

In January 2016, the US Department of Health & Human Services published new dietary guidelines. In their updated guidelines they recommend that added sugar consumption be limited to only ten percent or less of daily caloric intake.[101]

So that means that if you are on a 1500 calorie diet, you would consume a maximum of 150 calories from sugar.

While the guidelines address "added" sugar, they do not address naturally occurring sugars, such as those in fruit juice.

This is the first time that specific limits for added sugars have been included in the guidelines. "Because it's a new recommendation, and current food labels don't separate naturally occurring sugars from added sugars, some people may have difficulty discerning the difference between them, says Lisa Jones, MA, RDN, LDN, FAND, a spokesperson for the Pennsylvania Academy of Nutrition and Dietetics.[102]

"I think it's definitely a source of confusion," Jones says, adding that "information about added sugars currently isn't on food and beverage labels." The expectation is that added sugars will be included on food and beverage labels, but no changes [to labels] can be made until the FDA [issues its final ruling]." [103]

Jones says dietitians can help consumers better understand this guideline by putting it in context. She adds that many people are unaware of the amounts of added sugars in common foods. For example, many sodas, coffee-based drinks, and energy drinks can have significant amounts of added sugar.

---

[100] Tucker, ME. Sugar-Sweetened Beverages Linked to a Variety of Ills. *Medscape.* Oct 01, 2015. Accessed at: http://www.medscape.com/viewarticle/851956

[101] US Department of Health & Human Services. Dietary Guidelines for Americans 2015–2020: Eighth Edition. 2016, January 7. Published January 7, 2016. Accessed January 26, 2016 at: http://health.gov/dietaryguidelines/2015/guidelines/.

[102] Yeager, D. The 2015–2020 Dietary Guidelines. *Today's Dietitian.* 2016; 18(4)34. Accessed 9-05-16 at: http://www.todaysdietitian.com/newarchives/0416p34.shtml

[103] Yeager, D. The 2015–2020 Dietary Guidelines. *Today's Dietitian.* 2016; 18(4)34. Accessed 9-04-16 at: http://www.todaysdietitian.com/newarchives/0416p34.shtml

Although these drinks don't specifically list added sugars on their food labels, most of them certainly don't contain ingredients with naturally occurring sugars.

"In terms of translating the guideline for consumers, if you consider a 2,000 calorie diet, 10% of 2,000 calories equals 200 calories of added sugar. There are approximately 200 calories in 50g of sugar," Jones says. "If you look at sodas, there are approximately 35 g of sugar in a 12-oz can of soda, and that puts a person close to the recommended daily intake. Even non-soda beverages can have significant amounts of sugar, so it's still very important to read labels."[104]

If you want to *start* to get serious about the 10% rule, you might consider the naturally occurring sugars that are in so many foods.

And since the USDA guidelines address only *added* sugar, they don't address naturally occurring sugars. Food companies had been given until 2018 to list the added sugars on ingredient labels. But now the USDA went back on that promised deadline. Companies with $10,000,000 or more in sales must list added sugars beginning in 2020, while companies with less than $10,000,000 in sales now have until 2021 to comply. But that is just for added sugars. So we have to decide for ourselves the appropriate amount of sugar we will consume. And that goes for naturally occurring sugar as well as added sugar.

No matter the source of sugar, when that sugar gets into the bloodstream, blood sugar levels rise, and the pancreas releases insulin (or some may need to inject it). Do you think your body cares whether that increase in insulin levels is due to a natural response or a pharmaceutical injection? The fact is that when insulin is released into the bloodstream, it has the job of converting unused sugar into fat – to protect the body in case of famine. That is the job of insulin. Insulin opens the doors of our cells to accept glucose from our bloodstream. Whatever glucose our cells don't need for energy gets converted into fat for storage.

That's why it makes sense to count the grams of naturally occurring sugar in order to control blood sugar levels. Those natural sugars affect us just as much as added sugar.

And what about the information about the glycemic values of our foods that the World Health Organization recommends making available to consumers? Labeling our food with this information would show us which foods *quickly convert into sugar (glycose) during digestion.* It would also show us the effects

---

[104] Ibid.

of starchy foods that quickly convert into sugar during digestion. This crucial information is not accounted for when counting grams of sugar in a food, whether those sugars are naturally occurring or added. It will be much easier shopping if and when the information is made available on product packaging, and, of course must include labeling of GI information. But that still remains to be seen.

Surely it seems that nearly every individual sees the benefit of reducing the intake of added sugar. But this is not the case for food manufacturers. Added sugars are cheap, increase shelf life, create an addiction cycle [105] in the consumer, and add to the bottom line of food manufacturers, who also contribute significantly to political campaigns.

SAFETY IN NUMBERS

So, food manufacturers nearly began to be required to include labeling of any "added sugars" on their products in 2018. At that time they were also required to inform the public of the percent value of sugar their particular product will add to the daily diet. But that is not enough. Current labeling practices are still more about marketing than they are about nutrition.

Today, over twenty years after the World Health Organization recommended the use of the glycemic index be included in product labeling, we haven't even begun to label products with glycemic index in the USA. Glycemic index speaks for far more than "added sugar;" it also speaks for those foods that quickly convert into sugar through digestion and flood the body with glucose.

Only some of us know that added sugar is not the only aspect of a food that affects us. Many high starch foods like potatoes, cereals, and breads, for example, may not have natural or even added sugar, and can still have a far more powerful impact on us than natural or added sugar. Foods like Russet potatoes, pastas, rice, and processed grain products can and often do have a higher glycemic index than sucrose or even pure glucose.

But at least we'll finally begin to see the *added* sugar in a product.

And yet, regardless of all the labeling, marketing can't get around our sense of ourselves. We are the ones who can listen to the messages our body sends

[105] Lennerz B, Alsop D, Holsen L, et al. "Effects of dietary glycemic index on brain regions related to reward and craving Substance abuse and high-glycemic foods may trigger the same brain mechanism tied to addiction in men." Am J Clin Nutr, June 26, 2013 DOI: 10.3945/ajcn.113.064113. Accessed on 9-06-16 at: http://ajcn.nutrition.org/content/early/2013/06/26/ajcn.113.064113.abstract

out. All we have to do is notice. Just take the moment to check in with yourself – it's just one moment, and notice how you are feeling. That is being proactive. When we pay attention to how our body feels, how it reacts to certain foods, we can save our health. We CAN feel it when our body responds to food with a spike in blood sugar levels. We CAN feel it when our blood sugar levels fall and we get tired, crabby, and irritable. We just needed to know what to look out for, that's all. And don't expect to find it on a food label any time soon.

This is how we can reverse the progression of cardiovascular disease. This is how we can remain healthy and free of cancer. This is how we can avoid type 2 diabetes. This is how we can maintain stable blood glucose levels and our happy dispositions. This is the pathway to a long lifetime of health and happiness.

Consider that it took well over 30 years before the devillianization of fat in the diet even began as being the sole cause of cardiovascular disease. At that rate, do you think that glycemic index and glycemic load information will be readily available during your lifetime? Not if the arms of product marketing have anything to do with it. Do you want to wait until this information becomes mainstream (if it can ever break through profit driven marketing forces), or would you rather feel awesome for life starting right now?

Then you have to become aware of more than the potential roadblocks to managing the obvious sources of sugar consumption. The real question becomes, "how do we deal with sugars that are the result of quickly digested carbohydrates?" Here is when the glycemic index and glycemic load become the best friends you have ever had. They always tell you the truth because numbers do not lie.

SHOPPING FOR GROCERIES

❧ .... ❧

3 GROCERY SHOPPING TIPS

The best way to know what you need is to know what you already have on hand. Spending a few minutes taking stock can go a long way to save you money and allow you to build better meals.

1) Keep two lists posted on your refrigerator. They can be sticky notes or a note attached with a magnet.
   A. On the first list, write down ingredients you need to create recipes for your meals during the week. Add items you are low on or have run out of as that happens.
   B. You will use the second list when you come home from shopping. On the second list, keep track of the perishables such as fresh meat, fish, poultry, and produce you purchase or have on hand. Write down what it is and the expiration dates of items as you put them in the refrigerator. That way you will always know what you have on hand, and which you may want to use first.
2) Before you head to the store, using your phone, take a picture of the contents inside your fridge and pantry. This will serve as a good visual reminder while you shop.
3) Shop the peripheral of the store first, before going down any of the aisles. We will get into the details of this technique a bit later.

BECOMING A LABEL READER

We know that some foods, like whole fruits in their raw natural state, come with their own natural sugar. But most fruits also have fiber and other nutrients. Most fruits have a low glycemic index and/or glycemic load.

You can further learn of the glycemic index of specific foods in any of the International Tables of Glycemic Index and Glycemic Load through the links and references in this book.

Keep in mind that processing and cooking raises the glycemic index of foods. The more a food is processed, the higher the glycemic index becomes.

Chopping, grinding, "puffing," steaming, baking, roasting, shredding, boiling, baking, all break down fiber and expose more carbohydrate to the forces of digestion. These processes also lengthen the products' shelf life for the manufacturer. And all of these procedures raise the glycemic index for the consumer.

You can start by reading the labels on any packaged foods you use. When you are shopping for manufactured food products, you have to look beyond the "Food Facts" label. You have to read the very tiny print in the *ingredient list* to locate added sugars. An ingredient list is found on every manufactured food product. This is an additional list (much like a "supplement") to the more prominently displayed list of "Nutrition Facts" on these products. What you are looking for is in very fine print and begins with the heading "Ingredients:"

Once you find that list of ingredients, in order to recognize any added sugars, you have to know what you are looking for.

There are over 50 other names for "sugar." Manufacturers often spell added sugars to end with the letters "ose" or "rin" like dextrose or maltodextrin.

Here is a list to get you started in locating added sugars:

OVER 50 OTHER NAMES FOR SUGAR

1. Barley malt

2. Barbados sugar

3. Beet sugar

4. Brown sugar

5. Buttered syrup

6. Cane juice

7. Cane sugar

8. Caramel

9. Corn syrup

10. Corn syrup solids

11. Confectioner's sugar

12. Carob syrup

13. Castor sugar

14. Date sugar

15. Dehydrated cane juice

16. Demerara sugar

17. Dextran

18. Dextrose

19. Diastatic malt

20. Diatase

21. Ethyl maltol

22. Free Flowing Brown Sugars

23. Fructose

24. Fruit juice

25. Fruit juice concentrate

26. Galactose

27. Glucose

28. Glucose solids

29. Golden sugar

30. Golden syrup

31. Grape sugar

32. HFCS (High Fructose Corn Syrup)

33. Honey

34. Icing sugar

35. Invert sugar

36. Lactose

37. Malt

38. Maltodextrin

39. Maltose

40. Malt syrup

41. Mannitol

42. Maple syrup

43. Molasses

44. Muscovado

45. Panocha

46. Sor Ghum syrup

47. Crystalline fructose

48. Evaporated cane juice

49. Agave nectar

50. Treacle

51. Powdered sugar

52. Refiner's syrup

53. Rice syrup

54. Sorbitol

55. Erythritol

56. Xylitol –
57. Coconut Palm Sugar (GI of 45)

GETTING TO "NO SUGAR ADDED"

Beware of any product with added sugar, corn syrup, cane or rice syrup, corn sugar, honey, maple syrup, fructose, high fructose corn syrup (HFCS), fruit juice or fruit juice concentrate.

Look for any of the other names for sugar in the above list that may be included in the ingredient list on any product package.

That is, these are added sugars, in addition to any naturally occurring sugars.

Naturally occurring sugars that have high glycemic impact are in natural, even 100% natural and even organic fruit juices. Once the fruit is turned into a juice, it has lost most of its fiber. That fiber would have slowed down digestion. Our bodies digest liquids much faster than solids. Without fiber, that fruit juice has an impact much like sugar water.

Start by leaving these products at the store by at least one each week and you will help your overall health and improve your blood sugar levels. It will also help you overcome sugar addiction.

Be careful to read the ingredient labels of things you may least expect to contain processed sugars. Here is a roundup of some of the biggest culprits and their disguises:

- Fruit and vegetable "drinks"
- Manufactured sodas of any kind
- Coffee flavorings and "creamers" (on the shelves and also in the dairy section) and specialty coffee beverages
- Bread and bread products; bagels, donuts, muffins, pancakes, pizzas, pretzels, waffles
- Chips and crackers
- Candy
- Fruit and vegetable chips & dehydrated fruits and vegetables
- Yogurts and dairy products
- Pastas and rice
- Breakfast cereals in bags, boxes, and bulk
- Granola bars
- Dried fruits and fruit roll snacks
- Ready-made desserts of any kind
- Packaged cake mixes, pie crusts, cookie doughs
- Syrups, toppings, decorations

- Prepared sauces in cans and jars
- Dehydrated sauce mixes

Some of the items in the above list may have merely become habits in your shopping cart. Some of the items may be ingredients in some of your old familiar recipes. Shopping for those same old recipes and ingredients has become familiar. Familiarity is comfortable.

You take your shopping cart, and you go down the rows of the store, one at a time, and you place your selections into the cart. If other shoppers are blocking your way in the middle of an aisle, you glance at the shelves to see if there is another jar, box, or bag of something you can add to your cart. This way you haven't just wasted your time waiting for the other shoppers to pass. Just about every other shopper in the store shops this way too. Now, for your improved health, let's consider trying out a new technique. This can be a fun adventure.

PERIPHERAL SHOPPING

There is a much more exciting way to shop. And it nearly guarantees that you will check out of the store with much healthier food choices. It involves just a small change in habit.

The easiest way to change any habit is with new ideas. Everything starts with ideas. So here is a new and exciting idea for shopping:

Start your shopping by selecting items from the peripheral of the store. That's right, go around the whole store pushing your shopping cart in a big square along the outside aisles.

This is where you will find the fresh, live food items. You will note that the foods with the shortest shelf life are stocked here: fresh fruits and vegetables, fish, meat, and dairy products.

Start by looking at the fresh fruits and vegetables. Buy as many organic types as there are available. Consider ways to use these as the basis of some of your recipes.

Pretend for a few minutes that there are no inner aisles of the store, and that there are only these live fresh fruits and vegetables. Take a deep breath. Do you notice how clean the air is in the produce department? The tiny chloroplasts (plant cells) take in carbon dioxide and what we consider pollution and send out fresh oxygen into the air. The produce department is a wonderland of health. Enjoy your time here.

Celery sticks make a good replacement for chips. Carrots, broccoli, and cauliflower are also good choices.

Remember that image of the 8 cups of broccoli earlier in the book? Well how about finding a nice dip to create a side dish with some of the vegetables you like? Hummus makes a great dip and is available in a variety of flavors. Traditionally made with chick peas, it is now available in white bean varieties, too. Hummus is a delicious low glycemic option, either homemade or commercially prepared.

When you get to the fish, meat, and poultry department, try to select the freshest available. If you can find choices without antibiotics and growth hormones, those cuts are the best you can buy. You can think of it this way: The shorter the shelf life, the longer your life.

READING INGREDIENT LISTS – BRING A MAGNIFYING GLASS

After you circle the peripheral of the store filling your cart with fresh foods, you may find that you need some items located among the inner aisles. Just remember you will need to read the ingredient lists on everything that has a label. And don't think for a minute that just because a product has a name written in the largest bold print right on the front of it, that that name represents the main ingredient of that product.

Once you start reading ingredient labels, you will learn that many foods are not really what the bold print on their main labels claim that they are.

SUBSTITUTIONS FOR SUGAR

Watch out for products aimed at sugar replacement. For instance, many <u>Stevia</u> products are not mainly stevia at all. Even though the name on the product says it is "Stevia Extract," the label (in fine print) may say it is a "zero calorie liquid sweetener *made with Stevia extract.*"

Here is the list on one product that is boldly labeled as Stevia: Ingredients: water, erythritol, stevia extract, natural flavors, etc, etc, etc. This is true, even though the front of the container – in bold print – says that the product is Stevia.

But in this case, stevia is only the third ingredient listed on the product label. Products list their ingredients according to the order in which they occur. That means that there is more water and erythritol in that product than there is stevia.

Maybe you have already done some of your own research. Perhaps you have decided to use stevia extract instead of sugar because stevia doesn't raise blood sugar levels. If you have your heart set on natural stevia, one option is to get your own stevia plant at a gardening center. Take off a leaf or two to sweeten your beverage.

Or you might find some at a Health Food store. Real stevia extract is very concentrated. A single teaspoon of stevia extract delivers as much sweetness as an entire cup of sugar.

Erythritol is a sugar alcohol, also known as safe for blood glucose levels. But in order to discover that there is more erythritol than there is stevia in the product, you have to read such a tiny print list of ingredients. Better bring a magnifying glass with you whenever you shop in the center aisles of the grocery store.

Erythritol is manufactured by adding yeast to glucose. It does not promote tooth decay, nor does it cause gastric distress or bloating, and it has virtually no calories. Although it is less sweet, it also makes a good substitute for sugar, and it does not affect blood glucose levels.

Xylitol is another sugar alcohol. It has proven its ability to reduce dental carries, and even restore enamel to teeth. It has 33% fewer calories than table sugar, and does not raise blood glucose levels. The glycemic index of xylitol is only 7. It may cause gas and bloating in some people if eaten in excess. One word of caution: Xylitol can be deadly to animals, so be sure not to share with your pet.

IN CONCLUSION

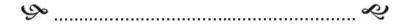

Harvard Medical School reports that "Glycemic index (GI) and glycemic load (GL) offer information about how foods affect blood sugar and insulin. The lower a food's glycemic index or glycemic load, the less it affects blood sugar and insulin levels." [106] They offer a list of over 100 foods and include the GI and the GL for each food on their website. You can follow the hyperlink or head over to the link in the footnotes to take a closer look at their list of foods.

 "The World Health Organization, American Diabetes Association, Diabetes UK, and Canadian Diabetes Association all give qualified support for the concept, yet, many health professionals consider the glycemic index and glycemic load to be too complex and too variable for use in clinical practice."[107]

How can we understand why there is so much resistance to using glycemic values? And what can we do to get the word out in ways that can help our brothers and sisters manage blood sugar levels?

It may be easy to understand why many healthcare professionals consider it too complex and too variable to use glycemic values in their practice, but it can save lives. Some patients may appreciate your simple recommendation, and go on to do some research on their own. Learning about creating resistant starch is an option that patients may easily understand. A good example of this might be the potato prep method we talked about earlier. It's something that can be used immediately.

Let's address the issues of "complexity" and "variability" right now. It certainly is a complex undertaking to collect and organize thousands of human test subjects, collect samples of thousands of foods from all over the world, conduct testing on human subjects, and finally to plot and organize test result data into one document. The sheer volume of data makes these international tables

---

[106]Harvard Medical School. "Glycemic index and glycemic load for 100+ foods." *Harvard Health Publications*. Updated Aug. 27, 2015. Retrieved from: http://www.health.harvard.edu/diseases-and-conditions/glycemic_index_and_glycemic_load_for_100_foods

[107] Atkinson FS, Foster-Powell K, Brand-Miller JC. "International tables of Glycemic Index and Glycemic Load Values: 2008." *Diabetes Care*. December; 31(12): 2281-2283. doi: 10.2337/dc08-1239 Retrieved from: http://www.ncbi.nlm.nih.gov/pmc/articles/PMC2584181/

complex. This requires a user to sort through a lot of data to find the information they are looking for.

As for *variability*, researchers compared test results of foods grown in soils of various countries and report the powerful effects of different soils, climates, and growing practices. Manipulating any of these factors can and does produce different and *variable* results.

So you will find countries of origin listed as well as preparation techniques for foods in the supplemental international tables of glycemic index and glycemic load. This also contributes to its complexity and variability. On the one hand, thank goodness we have access to all of this important information! On the other hand, can these international test result differences *really* be so great? Remember when we looked at the image comparing sweet potatoes and yams born in different countries earlier? Perhaps the next example will give us a better understanding of these issues.

In the next image we'll look at a comparison of five different foods born in the U.S.A. and those same foods born in Australia. The five foods in this example are Kellogg's All-Bran™, Special K™, Coca Cola®, Ocean Spray Cranberry Juice Cocktail®, and Sweet Corn. After the names and serving sizes of each of these 5 foods, you can see the side-by-side scientific test results for glycemic index (G.I.) and glycemic load (G.L.) in their respective columns:

COMPARISON:
SAME FOOD DIFFERENT COUNTRY

Food	Serving size	G. I. AUS	G. I. USA	G. L. AUS	G. L. USA
All-Bran™	30 g.	30	38	4	8
Special K™	30 g.	54	69	11	14
Coca Cola®	250 ml.	53	63	14	16
Ocean Spray Cranberry Juice Cocktail™	250 ml.	52	68	16	24
Sweet Corn	80 g.	48	60	8	11

G.I. AUS = Glycemic Index in Australia
G.I. USA = Glycemic Index in USA
G.L. AUS = Glycemic Load in Australia
G.L. USA = Glycemic Load in USA

[108]

By comparing the food test results in the above table, you may notice that the same foods born in Australia have a lower glycemic index and glycemic load when tested using human subjects than those same foods born in the United States of America. This is why consumers need country specific glycemic index scores.

Australia and New Zealand include the GI on their food labels. This information guides consumer purchases. It also offers feedback to those responsible for manufacturing procedures. This may lead to adjustments in growing practices, and certainly to amounts of certain recipe ingredients that could be used to create more healthful products.

[108] Atkinson F, Foster-Powell K, Brand-Miller J. "International tables of Glycemic Index and Glycemic Load Values: 2008." *Diabetes Care*. December; 31(12): 2281-2283. Doi: 10.2337/dc08-1239. Retrieved from: http://www.ncbi.nlm.nih.gov/pmc/articles/PMC2584181/

Yet, even plain fresh sweet corn has a lower GI and GL in Australia than it does in the U.S.A. Perhaps this is a good example of the effects of different growing practices. As we discussed, there are a multitude of possible reasons.

The U.S.A. has chosen not to subscribe to the recommendations of the Food and Agriculture Organization of the United Nations or the World Health Organization. Unfortunately, GI food labeling is not currently being practiced in the U.S.A. As a result, the potential feedback loop is missing for food manufacturers, farmers, and even recipe creators. In most countries, consumers have to discover on their own that there even is such a thing as a glycemic index!

It is not the fault of our healthcare providers, or the media who deluge us with commercials for those "endless fries," or even the American Diabetes Association for their inaccurate information. The information certainly is complex, and it is definitely variable from country to country.

We may begin to understand that the abuse of carbohydrate begins with quicker-to-harvest growing practices, continues by over-processing and "refining" our foods, and finishes by manufacturing and "enrichment" to produce "food-like" products many have grown to depend on.

The processing of any natural, whole foods gives them a higher glycemic index than their non-processed counterparts. This is because the high carbohydrate endosperm portion forms the bulk of a product, and the fiber (bran) is also broken down or in many cases, totally removed.

To help our bodies deal with some starchy foods we've looked at the preparation technique of creating resistant starch. This lowers glycemic index of many foods, as demonstrated in the results of the international tables. We've also looked at adjusting serving sizes to lower the glycemic load, another important factor in blood sugar control.

How can consumers find out about all of this crucial information? The most up-to-date information is available at no cost through our National Institutes of Health.[109] Originally published by Diabetes Care, this life-changing information is just waiting to be discovered. A second option is to go to

---

[109] Atkinson F, Foster-Powell K, Brand-Miller J. "International tables of Glycemic Index and Glycemic Load Values: 2008." *Diabetes Care*. December; 31(12): 2281-2283. Doi: 10.2337/dc08-1239. Retrieved from: http://www.ncbi.nlm.nih.gov/pmc/articles/PMC2584181/

http://www.glycemicindex.com/[110] and search the online database at the University of Sydney for any food entry.

When we take advantage of the opportunity to work with glycemic values, we can take control of the destiny of our health, both mental and physical. This natural way to blood sugar control avoids blood sugar spikes, crashes, and the resulting diseases and disorders they create. This is a powerful tool we can use to improve our own health and lifespan. And it may help us bring change to the lives of those we touch. We're all in this together.

Thank you for taking your time to read this book. I know it contains a lot of information.

With any luck, you may recognize why glycemic values are worth exploring and incorporating into your food selection process. If you are convinced that it's worth it, that is reward enough for me. And for those of you who succeed at keeping a low glycemic load lifestyle, the results shown on your annual physical exam may be reward enough for you!

APPENDIX:
PERSONAL GLYCEMIC LOAD WORKBOOK & TABLE

℘ .... ℘

USING YOUR GLYCEMIC LOAD WORKBOOK

I t might be best to use a pencil when entering your data into the pages of the Glycemic Load Workbook (pg. 110 – 123). This way you'll be able to erase and re-enter different serving sizes, available carbs, and GL, depending on the amount of each food that you eat. Maintaining a Glycemic Load of 10 or less is the key to success.

If you are working from the Print Replica version, you may want to make notes or highlights in the book, or take some notes on paper so you have a reference to look back on as you progress. A sheet of notebook and a ruler will help you create just what you need. This will help you keep track of the information that is pertinent to you. When you determine a low glycemic load serving of any food in your Glycemic Load Workbook, you have created one little resource. You're off to a great start!

Using the Glycemic Load Workbook, determine the best serving sizes of other foods you enjoy often. When you establish low glycemic load serving sizes, copy this information (Food, GI, Serv size, Available Carbs, and GL) to a Personal Glycemic Load Table (pgs. 124-128), or make your own table on paper. As you continue to calculate low glycemic load servings of other foods you frequently enjoy in the Workbook, copy the information to your Personal Glycemic Load Table. Continue in this manner until you have gathered the data for all the foods in your life. The Workbook and Personal Table become your own personalized references to keep track of your mastery of using glycemic load.

Watch it grow as the Personal Glycemic Load Table becomes your own individualized "Cheat Sheet." You may cut your Personal Glycemic Load Table from the book if you like and take it along with you wherever you go.

Here's the step-by-step process from the beginning:

1. GI: Select a food or beverage listed in the "FOOD" section of the Workbook. Notice the GI of that food. The GI of a food always stays the same. If the food you select has a GI of "0," no serving

size is required because that food does not affect blood sugar levels no matter the serving size. Enter it in your Personal Table.

2. Serv Size: In the next column, marked "Serv Size", enter the amount you plan to eat. You may use Metric or Customary US measures for your serving size.

3. Avail Carbs: Determine the Available Carbohydrate for your chosen serving size. This is the total carbohydrate minus the amount of Fiber in your serving. See "Nutrition Fact" labels, or the USDA National Nutrient Database at Food Data Central.[111] Enter the Available Carbohydrate in the "Avail Carbs" column, right next to the Serv Size for that food.

4. GL: Calculate the GL as we discussed in the book. Enter the Glycemic Load for your serving size in the column marked "GL." When it is 10 or less, you have selected a low glycemic load serving. Good job! Congratulations! If it is over 10, you can adjust the serving size down, or possibly substitute a food with a lower Glycemic Index.

5. Copy the information into your Personal Glycemic Load Table.

Here is the calculation again:

(Available) Carbohydrate X Glycemic Index = _____ / 100 = Glycemic Load

The "Glycemic Load Workbook with Glycemic Index for Over 350 Foods" is in alphabetical order. It lists the Glycemic Index of each food or beverage. The majority of entries are from subjects with normal glucose tolerance, but also includes some food entries with results on type 2 diabetics or those with impaired glucose tolerance. These types of test subjects are mentioned in parentheses following the names of the foods in the FOOD column entries.

You will also find some results for different preparation and serving techniques in the table that have a scientifically proven ability to lower the glycemic index (GI) of some foods. These entries include the words "Special Prep" underlined in the food description. (Whenever you lower the GI of a food, the glycemic load [GL] naturally becomes lower as well.) Finally, if available, the manufacturer and/or country that sponsored the testing of that food is listed in parentheses at the end of that food entry as well.

---

[111] https://fdc.nal.usda.gov/

GLYCEMIC LOAD WORKBOOK WITH GLYCEMIC INDEX FOR OVER 350 FOODS

FOOD	GI	Serv Size	Avail Carbs	GL
Almond meal flour	0			
Almond Milk, unsweetened	0			
Almonds	0			
Animal protein, including wild game	0			
Apple juice, unsweetened	41			
Apple juice, unsweetened	40			
Apple muffin, made with rolled oats and sugar	44			
Apple muffin, made with rolled oats and without sugar	48			
Apple slices with peanut butter	38			
Apples, raw, type not specified	40			
Apricots, raw	40			
Artichoke	40			
Arugula	40			
Asparagus	40			
Avocado	0			
Banana, raw, average (in type 2 Diabetics)	47			
Barley, Pearled, average	25			
Beans, baked	40			
Beans, Black (Wil-Pack Foods, San Pedro, CA.)	64			
Beans, Black, boiled	30			
Beans, Chickpeas, boiled	10			
Beans, Chickpeas, canned in brine	42			
Beans, Kidney, boiled	34			
Beans, Lentils, boiled	29			
Beans, Navy, average, boiled	39			
Beans, Pinto, boiled in salted water	14			
Beans, Soy Beans, boiled	15			
Beet greens	40			
Bell pepper	40			
Blackberries	0			
Blueberries	29			
Bok Choy	40			
Boysenberries	40			
Bread, 100% Whole Grain™ (Natural Ovens, USA)	51			
Bread, 50% cracked wheat kernel	58			

FOOD	GI	Serv Size	Avail Carbs	GL
Bread, Bagel, white (USA)	69			
Bread, Bagel, white, frozen	72			
Bread, Baguette, white, plain	93			
Bread, Coarse barley, 80% kernels	34			
Bread, English Muffin™ (Natural Ovens USA)	77			
Bread, Hamburger bun	61			
Bread, Happiness™ (cinnamon raisin pecan bread) (Natural Ovens Manitowoc USA)	63			
Bread, Healthy Choice™ Hearty 100% Whole Grain (Con Agra Inc. USA)	62			
Bread, Healthy Choice™ Hearty 7 Grain (Con Agra Inc. USA)	55			
Bread, Hunger Filler™ Whole Grain (Natural Ovens USA)	59			
Bread, Kaiser roll	73			
Bread, made with Whole-meal (whole-wheat) wheat-flour (USA)	73			
Bread, Muesli bread made from packet mix in bread making machine (Con Agra Inc. USA)	54			
Bread, Nutty Natural™ whole grain bread (Natural Ovens USA)	59			
Bread, Pita white	68			
Bread, Pumpernickel	56			
Bread, Rye kernel, 80% kernels	55			
Bread, Soy & Linseed bread (made from packet mix, cooked in bread maker) (Con Agra Inc. USA)	50			
Bread, Special prep: 30 g. white bread served with 51 g. baked beans (UK)	50			
Bread, Special prep: 30 g. white bread, toasted, served with 36 g. cheddar cheese (UK)	35			
Bread, Special prep: White bread, prepared with a 10 min. prove and a second 2 min. prove (low volume loaf) (UK)	50			
Bread, Special prep: White wheat flour bread, toasted	50			
Bread, Special prep: White wheat flour bread, toasted, mean of 3 studies (UK)	60			
Bread, Special Prep: White wheat flour	75			

FOOD	GI	Serv Size	Avail Carbs	GL
bread, frozen, defrosted (British Bakeries, Ltd. UK)				
Bread, Special Prep: White wheat flour bread, frozen, defrosted, and toasted (British Bakeries, Ltd. UK	64			
Bread, Stay Trim™ whole grain bread (Natural Ovens USA)	70			
Bread, White wheat flour, average	75			
Bread, White wheat flour, white flour (Pepperidge Farm Norwalk CT USA)	71			
Bread, whole wheat, average	71			
Bread, Wonder® bread, enriched white bread (Interstate Brands Companies, Kansas City, MO, USA) Mean of 3 studies	73			
Broccoli	40			
Bulgur, average, cooked	47			
Cabbage	40			
Cake, Arepa, corn bread cake, made with corn flour (Mexico)	72			
Cake, Arepa, made from dehulled high-amylose (70%) corn flour	44			
Cake, Arepa, made from ordinary dehulled dent corn flour (25% amylose)	81			
Cake, Banana, made with sugar	47			
Cake, Banana, made without sugar	55			
Cake, Chocolate Raspberry Ganache cupcakes (From recipe in Are You Sweet Enough Already?)	35			
Cake, Chocolate, made from packet mix with chocolate frosting (Betty Crocker General Mills Inc. Minneapolis USA)	38			
Cake, Sponge	46			
Cake, Vanilla, made from packet mix with vanilla frosting (Betty Crocker USA)	42			
Cantaloupe	40			
Carob powder, unsweetened	40			
Carrots, average	39			
Cashews	22			
Cauliflower	40			
Celery	40			

FOOD	GI	Serv Size	Avail Carbs	GL
Celery with Cashew Butter	40			
Celery with Hummus	40			
Cereal, All-Bran™, average, (Kellogg's, Battle Creek, MI, USA) (in normal individuals)	47			
Cereal, Cornflakes (Kellogg's, USA)	92			
Cereal, Grapenuts (Kraft Foods Inc, Port Chester, NY, USA)	75			
Cereal, Hot, apple & cinnamon (Con Agra Inc USA)	37			
Cereal, Hot, apple and cinnamon (Con Agra Inc, USA)	37			
Cereal, Hot, unflavored (Con Agra Inc, USA)	25			
Cereal, Hot, unflavored (Con Agra Inc. USA)	25			
Cereal, Kashi Seven Whole Grain Puffs®	65			
Cereal, Oats, instant, average, one packet (41g) prepared with water	79			
Cereal, Oats, Porridge, make from steel cut oats boiled in water	52			
Cereal, Raisin Bran (Kellogg's, USA)	61			
Cereal, Special K® (Kellogg's, USA)	69			
Cherries, red	40			
Chicken nuggets, frozen, reheated in microwave 5 min.	46			
Chickpea flour	10			
Chocolate dark Dove® (M&M/Mars USA)	23			
Chocolate weight management bar (Shaklee Corporation Pleasanton, CA USA)	29			
Choicedm™ vanilla (Mead Johnson Nutritionals Evansville USA)	23			
Cinch™ Café Latte weight management powder prepared with skim milk (Shaklee Corporation Pleasanton USA)	27			
Cinch™ Chocolate weight management powder prepared with skim milk (Shaklee Corporation USA)	16			
Cinch™ Vanilla weight management powder prepared with skim milk	22			

FOOD	GI	Serv Size	Avail Carbs	GL
Clif bar Chocolate Brownie Energy bar (Clif Bar Inc. Berkeley USA)	57			
Coca Cola®	63			
Cocoa powder, unsweetened	40			
Cocoavia™ Chocolate Almond Snack bar (M&M/Mars USA)	63			
Cocoavia™ Crispy Chocolate Bar (M&M/Mars USA)	33			
Coconut flour	42			
Coconut Milk, unsweetened	40			
Coffee or tea, black, unsweetened	0			
Collard greens	40			
Combos Snacks Cheddar Cheese Crackers (M&M/Mars USA)	54			
Combos Snacks Cheddar Cheese Pretzels (M&M/Mars USA)	52			
Cookies, Ranger Cookies (From recipe in *Are You Sweet Enough Already?*)	35			
Cookies, Shortbread	64			
Cookies, Vanilla wafers	77			
Corn chips	42			
Corn, Popcorn, microwave, plain, average	55			
Corn, Sweet corn (USA)	60			
Corn, Sweet corn on the cob	48			
Corn, Sweet corn, whole-kernel, diet pack, Featherweight™, canned, drained, heated, (USA)	46			
Cranberries	40			
Cranberry juice cocktail (Ocean Spray Inc., USA)	68			
Creamed cottage cheese	30			
Cucumber	40			
Dandelion greens	40			
Dates	42			
Dill Pickle	40			
Egg, hardboiled	0			
Eggplant	40			
Enercal Plus, made from powder (Wyeth-Ayerst International Inc, Madison, NJ, US)	61			
Enercal Plus™, made from powder (Wyeth-Ayerst International Inc	61			

FOOD	GI	Serv Size	Avail Carbs	GL
Madison USA)				
Ensure Pudding, old-fashioned vanilla (Abbott Laboratories Inc, Ashland, OH, USA)	36			
ExtendBar™ Apple Cinnamon Delight Bar (USA)	33			
ExtendBar™ Chocolate Delight Bar (USA)	41			
ExtendBar™ Peanut Delight Bar (USA)	32			
Fanta®	68			
Fats and Oils	0			
Figs	40			
Fruit punch (USA)	67			
Fruit roll-Ups®	99			
Garlic	40			
Gatorade®, orange flavor	89			
Ginger root	40			
Glucerna diabetes-specific enteral formula Abbott Laboratories Inc USA)	15			
Glucerna SR diabetes-specific enteral formula (Abbott Laboratories Inc. USA)	23			
Glucerna™ vanilla (Abbott Laboratories Inc. USA)	31			
Graham crackers	74			
Grape leaves	40			
Grapefruit	25			
Grapes, Black	59			
Green beans	40			
Green Leaf Lettuce	0			
Green peas, average	54			
Guava	40			
Hazelnuts	0			
Honeydew	40			
Hummus (chickpea salad dip), commercially prepared	6			
Ice cream, premium (Sara Lee®)	38			
Ice cream, regular, average	62			
Ironman PR bar® chocolate (PR Nutrition San Diego CA USA)	39			
Jicama	40			
Kale	40			
Kiwi	40			
Kohlrabi	40			

FOOD	GI	Serv Size	Avail Carbs	GL
Kudos Milk Chocolate Granola bar with M&M's Milk Chocolate Mini Baking Bits (M&M/Mars USA)	52			
Kudos Milk Chocolate Granola bars Peanut Butter flavor (M&M/Mars USA)	45			
Kudos Whole-Grain Bars, chocolate chip (M& M/Mars, Hackettstown, NJ, USA)	62			
L.E.A.N (Life long) Nutribar, chocolate crunch	32			
L.E.A.N (Life long) Nutribar, peanut crunch	30			
L.E.A.N Fibergy bar, harvest oat	45			
Leek	40			
Lemon weight management bar (Shaklee Corporation USA)	23			
Lychee	40			
M&M's®, peanut	33			
Macadamia nuts	0			
Mandarin	40			
Mango	40			
Mars Active® Energy Drink flavored milk (M&M/Mars USA)	46			
Mars Bar® (M&M/Mars USA)	68			
Milk skim (USA)	32			
Milk, skim, average	31			
Milky Way® bar (M&M/Mars USA)	62			
Milky Way® Lite bar (M&M/Mars USA)	45			
Mulberries	40			
Munch Peanut Butter bar (M&M/Mars USA)	27			
Mushrooms	40			
Mustard greens	40			
Nopal (prickly pear cactus)	7			
Nutrimeal™ meal replacement drink Dutch Chocolate (Usana, Salt Lake City, USA)	26			
Okra	40			
Olives	40			
Onion	40			
Orange juice, reconstituted from frozen concentrate (USA)	57			
Orange juice, unsweetened	50			

FOOD	GI	Serv Size	Avail Carbs	GL
Orange, raw (Sunkist, Van Nuys, CA, USA)	48			
Papaya	40			
Parsnips	52			
Passionfruit	40			
Pasta, Fettucine	32			
Pasta, Macaroni and Cheese (Kraft®)	64			
Pasta, Macaroni, average	50			
Pasta, Proti pasta protein-enriched boiled in water (Vital Nature Inc San Antonio TX USA)	28			
Pasta, Spaghetti, white, boiled 20 min.	58			
Pasta, Spaghetti, white, Durum wheat, boiled 20 min (USA)	58			
Pasta, Spaghetti, whole meal, boiled (USA)	32			
Pasta, Spaghetti, whole-grain, boiled	42			
Peach, average	42			
Peaches, canned in light syrup	52			
Peanut Butter weight management bar (Shaklee Corporation USA)	22			
Peanuts	7			
Pear	38			
Pear, canned in pear juice	44			
Pecans	0			
Performance Chocolate Energy bar (Power Bar USA) Power Bar® (Powerfood Inc. Berkeley USA)	53			
Persimmon	40			
Pineapple	40			
Pirate's Booty aged white cheddar extruded snack made from corn and rice (Robert's American Gourmet Sea Cliff NY USA)	70			
Pizza, plain baked dough, served with parmesan cheese and tomato sauce	80			
Pizza, Super Supreme (Pizza Hut®)	36			
Plantain	40			
Plum	40			
Pomegranate	40			
Potato chips, average	56			
Potato, baked russet	111			
Potato, boiled in salted water (India)	76			

FOOD	GI	Serv Size	Avail Carbs	GL
Potato, French fries (Ore Ida Golden Fries)	64			
Potato, instant mashed, average	88			
Potato, Red, boiled with skin on in salted water for 12 min (Canada)	89			
Potato, Red, cubed, Special prep, boiled in salted water 12 min, stored overnight in refrigerator, consumed cold (Canada)	56			
Potato, Russet Burbank, baked without fat, 45–60 min (USA) (in type 2 Diabetics)	78			
Potato, Russet, baked without fat (USA) (in normal individuals)	111			
Potato, Russet, baked without fat (USA) (in type 2 Diabetics or those with impaired glucose tolerance)	94			
Potato, Sava, peeled, boiled 21-30 min (Sweden)	118			
Potato, Sava, peeled, boiled 21-30 min, refrigerated 24 h, consumed cold (Sweden)	88			
Potato, Sava, Special prep, peeled, boiled 21-30 min, refrigerated 24 h, consumed cold with white vinegar (28 g) and olive oil (8g) (Sweden)	67			
Potato, Special prep. boiled in salted water, refrigerated, reheated (India)	23			
Potato, sweet, average	70			
Potato, white, boiled, average	82			
Potato, yam, average	54			
Pretzels, oven-baked	83			
Promote with fiber™ nutritional supplement (Ross Nutrition USA)	49			
Prunes, pitted	29			
Quinoa	53			
Radicchio	40			
Radish	40			
Raisins	64			
Raspberries	0			
Rhubarb	40			
Rice cakes, average	82			
Rice, Brown & Wild Uncle Ben's®	45			

FOOD	GI	Serv Size	Avail Carbs	GL
Ready Whole Grain Medley™ (pouch) (Effem Foods USA)				
Rice, Brown Rice Uncle Ben's® Ready Whole Grain (pouch) (Effem Foods USA)	48			
Rice, Brown, steamed (USA)	50			
Rice, Chicken Flavored Brown Rice Uncle Ben's® Ready Whole Grain (pouch) (Effem Foods USA)	46			
Rice, Converted, white, boiled 20–30 min (Uncle Ben's; Masterfoods USA, Vernon, CA)	38			
Rice, Converted, white, long grain, boiled 20–30 min (Uncle Ben's; Masterfoods USA)	50			
Rice, Long Grain and Wild Uncle Ben's® Ready Rice (pouch) (Effem Foods USA)	49			
Rice, Original Long Grain Uncle Ben's® Ready Rice (pouch) (Effem Foods USA)	48			
Rice, Parboiled (USA)	72			
Rice, Special Prep, Parboiled (Uncle Ben's Converted, consumed with 68 g cheese and 14 g butter (Uncle Ben's Converted, Mars, USA.) (Canada)	27			
Rice, Roasted Chicken Flavored, Uncle Ben's® Ready (pouch) Effem Foods USA)	51			
Rice, Santa Fe Uncle Ben's® Ready Whole Grain Medley™ (pouch) (Effem Foods USA)	48			
Rice, Spanish Style Uncle Ben's® Ready Rice pouch) (Effem Foods USA)	51			
Rice, Vegetable Harvest Uncle Ben's® Ready Whole Grain Medley™ (pouch) (Effem Foods USA)	48			
Rice, White, boiled	72			
Rice, white, quick cooking Basmati	63			
Rose hips	40			
Rye crisps, average	64			
Seltzer water, baking extract flavored, stevia sweetened	0			

FOOD	GI	Serv Size	Avail Carbs	GL
Slim Fast™ French Vanilla ready-to-drink shake (Slim Fast Foods Company Englewood USA)	37			
Slimfast® Meal Options bar rich chocolate brownie (SlimFast Foods Co West Palm Beach USA)	64			
SmartZone Nutrition Bar Chocolate flavor (Hershey's® Foods Corp. Hershey PA, USA.)	11			
SmartZone Nutrition Bar Chocolate flavor (Hershey's®, USA.)	16			
SmartZone Nutrition Bar Crunchy Blueberry flavor (Hershey's® USA.)	15			
SmartZone Nutrition Bar Crunchy Chocolate Brownie flavor (Hershey's® USA.)	23			
SmartZone Nutrition Bar Crunchy Chocolate Caramel flavor (Hershey's® USA.)	16			
SmartZone Nutrition Bar Crunchy Chocolate Peanut Butter flavor (Hershey's® USA.)	14			
SmartZone Nutrition Bar Crunchy Key Lime flavor (Hershey's® USA.)	14			
SmartZone Nutrition Bar Peanut Butter flavor Snickers® Marathon Energy Bar (Hershey's® USA)	18			
Smoothie banana & strawberry V8 Splash® (Campbell's Soup Co Camden USA)	44			
Smoothie raspberry (Con Agra Inc Omaha USA)	33			
Snack bar Apple Cinnamon (Con Agra Inc. Omaha NE USA)	40			
Snack bar Peanut Butter and Choc-Chip (Con Agra Inc. USA)	37			
Snickers Bar®, average	51			
Snickers® (M&M/Mars, USA) Marathon Nutrition Bar Dark Chocolate Crunch flavor	49			
Snickers® (M&M/Mars, USA)Marathon Energy Bar Cookies & Crème flavor	50			
Snickers® Marathon Energy Bar Chewy	36			

FOOD	GI	Serv Size	Avail Carbs	GL
Chocolate Peanut flavor (M&M/Mars, USA)				
Snickers® Marathon Energy Bar Multi Grain Crunch flavor (M&M/Mars, USA)	50			
Snickers® Marathon Energy Bar Peanut Butter flavor (M&M/Mars, USA)	34			
Snickers® Marathon Low Carb Lifestyle Energy Bar Chocolate Fudge Brownie flavor (M&M/Mars, USA)	20			
Snickers® Marathon Low Carb Lifestyle Energy Bar Peanut Butter flavor (M&M/Mars, USA)	21			
Snickers® Marathon Nutrition Bar Honey & Roasted Almond flavor (M&M/Mars, USA)	41			
Snickers® Marathon Protein Performance Bar (M&M/Mars, USA) Caramel Nut Rush flavor	26			
Snickers® Marathon Protein Performance Bar Chocolate Nut Burst flavor (M&M/Mars, USA)	32			
Soda crackers	74			
Soup, Black Bean (Wil-Pack Foods, San Pedro, CA, USA)	64			
Soup, Minestrone, condensed, prepared with water (Campbell's Soup Company Camden NJ USA)	48			
Soup, Split Pea (Wil-Pak Foods, USA)	60			
Soup, Tomato, condensed, prepared with water (Campbell's Soup Company Camden NJ USA)	52			
Soursop	40			
Soy protein chips, "Sunshine"™ lightly salted, (Revival Soy®Physicians Pharmaceuticals Inc. USA)	87			
Spinach	0			
Strawberries	40			
Strawberry fruit leather (Stretch Island Fruit Company™ Washington USA)	29			
Sweetener, Blackstrap molasses	55			
Sweetener, Coconut palm sugar	35			
Sweetener, Fructose, 50g. (Sigma Chemical Co., St. Louis, MO, USA)	24			
Sweetener, Honey, Buckwheat, ratio of	73			

FOOD	GI	Serv Size	Avail Carbs	GL
fructose: glucose 1.12 (Vazza Farms USA)				
Sweetener, Honey, Clover, ratio of fructose: glucose 1.09 (Vazza Farms Hermiston OR USA)	69			
Sweetener, Honey, Premium Agave nectar (Sweet Cactus Farms USA), mean of three studies	19			
Sweetener, Honey, Tupelo, ratio of fructose: glucose 1.54 (Tropical Blossom Honey Co Edgewater FL USA)	74			
Sweetener, Lactose, 50g. (Sigma Chemical Co., USA	43			
Sweetener, Stevia extract	0			
Sweetener, Stevia packet	0			
Sweetener, Sucrose, 50g. (Sigma Chemical Co. USA)	58			
Sweetener, Xylitol (1 packet)	7			
Swiss chard	40			
Tangerine	40			
Tofu-based frozen dessert, chocolate with high fructose (24%) corn syrup (USA)	115			
Tomatillo	40			
Tomato	40			
Tomato juice, canned	38			
Tortilla, Corn (Mexican)	52			
Tortilla, Corn, fried, with mashed potato, fresh tomato and lettuce (Mexican)	78			
Tortilla, Corn, served with refried mashed pinto beans and tomato sauce (Mexican)	39			
Tortilla, Wheat (Mexican)	30			
Tortilla, Wheat, served with refried pinto beans and tomato sauce (Mexican)	28			
Turmeric root	40			
Twix® Cookie Bar caramel (M&M/Mars USA)	44			
Ultracal™ with fiber (Mead Johnson, USA)	40			
Usana L.E.A.N (Life long) Nutribar™ Chocolate Crunch (Usana Inc, Salt	32			

FOOD	GI	Serv Size	Avail Carbs	GL
Lake City, UT, US)				
Usana L.E.A.N (Life long) Nutribar™ Peanut Crunch (Usana Inc, Salt Lake City, UT, US)	30			
Usana L.E.A.N Fibergy™ bar Harvest Oat (Usana Inc, Salt Lake City, UT, US)	45			
Usana Nutrimeal™ meal replacement drink powder Dutch Chocolate (Usana Inc, Salt Lake City, UT, US)	26			
V8 Splash® tropical blend fruit drink (Campbell's Soup Company USA)	47			
V8® 100% vegetable juice (Campbell's Soup Company USA)	43			
VO2 Max Chocolate Energy bar (M&M/Mars USA)	49			
Waffles, Aunt Jemima®	76			
Walnuts	0			
Water	0			
Watercress	40			
Watermelon	72			
Wheatgrass	40			
ZonePerfect® Nutrition bar Double Chocolate flavor (Abbott Laboratories Abbott Park USA)	44			
Zucchini	40			

[112], [113], [114]

[112] Atkinson F, Foster-Powell K, Brand-Miller J. "International tables of Glycemic Index and Glycemic Load Values: 2008." *Diabetes Care*. December; 31(12): 2281-2283. Doi: 10.2337/dc08-1239. Retrieved from: http://www.ncbi.nlm.nih.gov/pmc/articles/PMC2584181/

[113] http://www.glycemicindex.com/

[114] http://www.health.harvard.edu/diseases-and-conditions/glycemic_index_and_glycemic_load_for_100_foods

PERSONAL GLYCEMIC LOAD TABLE

FOOD	GI	Serv Size	Avail Carbs	GL

FOOD	GI	Serv Size	Avail Carbs	GL

FOOD	GI	Serv Size	Avail Carbs	GL

FOOD	GI	Serv Size	Avail Carbs	GL

OTHER BOOKS BY THIS AUTHOR

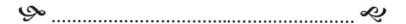

Cheat Sheet Simply for USA Foods includes scientifically tested results for over 375 foods born in the U.S.A. Includes tables of Glycemic Index, Carbohydrate, Fiber, and Glycemic Load for typical serving sizes. With complete overview of using glycemic values for food selection.

Cheat Sheet Simply for UK Foods includes scientifically tested results for 390 foods born in the United Kingdom of Great Britain. Includes tables of Glycemic Index, Carbohydrate, Fibre, and Glycemic Load for typical serving sizes. With complete overview of using glycemic values for food selection.

Cheat Sheet Simply for Canadian Foods includes scientifically tested results over 475 foods born in Canada. Includes tables of Glycemic Index, Carbohydrate, Fiber, and Glycemic Load for typical serving sizes. With complete overview of using glycemic values for food selection.

Triche Feuille Simplement Pour Les Aliments Français alec plus de 335 aliments nés en France. Comprend des tableaux d'index glycémique, de glucides, de fibres et de charge glycémique pour les portions typiques. Avec un aperçu complet de l'utilisation des valeurs glycémiques pour la sélection des aliments. (Cheat Sheet Simply for French Foods with over 335 foods born in France.)

Fat Facts: Optimize Your Atkins, Glycemic Index, Low-Carb, Keto, or Paleo Diet to Lose Weight, Reverse Disease, Boost Brain Health, and Increase Lifespan. Includes nutrition facts on the content of dietary fats.

Nutrient Essentials details the essential healing nutrients that must be supplied by our diets. Includes tables of dietary fats and foods with macronutrient content for typical serving sizes. With guidance on essential Amino Acids and Vitamins B. Includes resources for lactose intolerance, minerals for retaining bone strength (and those to avoid), and menopause support.

Are You Sweet Enough Already? 10 Low Glycemic Load Desserts for Blood Sugar Control. Complete with overview of using glycemic values. These recipes include nutrition data including Glycemic Index (GI), Glycemic load (GL) per serving, calories, protein, carbohydrate, fiber, fat, saturated fat, and sodium per serving.

Low Glycemic Happiness 120 Recipes for Blood Sugar Control, with Dr. Maury Breecher. These recipes include nutrition data including Glycemic Index (GI), Glycemic load (GL) per serving, calories, protein, carbohydrate, fiber, fat, saturated fat, and sodium per serving.

Beyond the Knife, Alternatives to Surgery, with Alan Lazar, MD, FACS, and Dr. Maury Breecher PhD, MPH. Many alternatives for those who prefer natural healing over surgery.

Made in the USA
Columbia, SC
11 February 2021

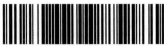